Cooper Gets An X-ray

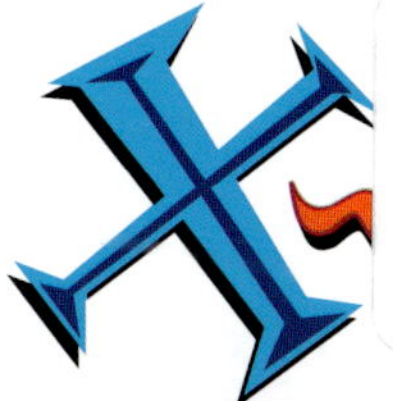

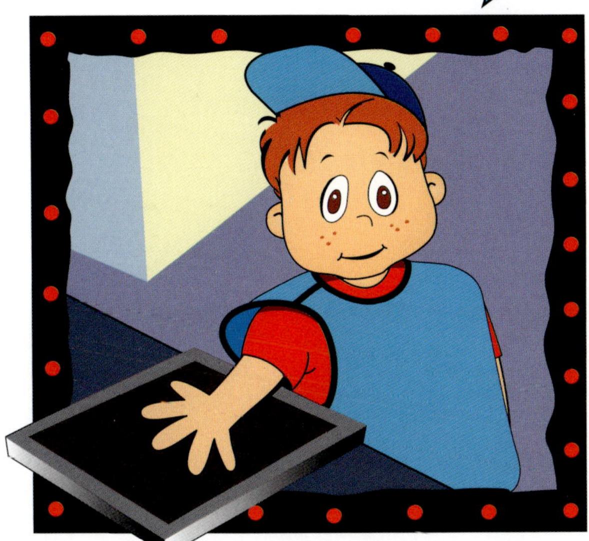

Cooper shares his
experience of having an X-ray, so
other children can learn this simple
medical procedure.

Created & Written by Karen Olson

Illustrated by Joanne Kollman

Graphic Design by Nangeroni Designs

Edited by Ellie Martin

~ Special Acknowledgements ~

Peggy Adams • Child Life Coordinator
Claire Bettlestone • Diagnostic Radiologist
Connie Brandenburg • CT Coordinator
Donald Craig, MD • Associate Clinical Professor of Pediatrics
Christine Lolich, RN, BS • Manager of Adult & Children's Emergency Departments

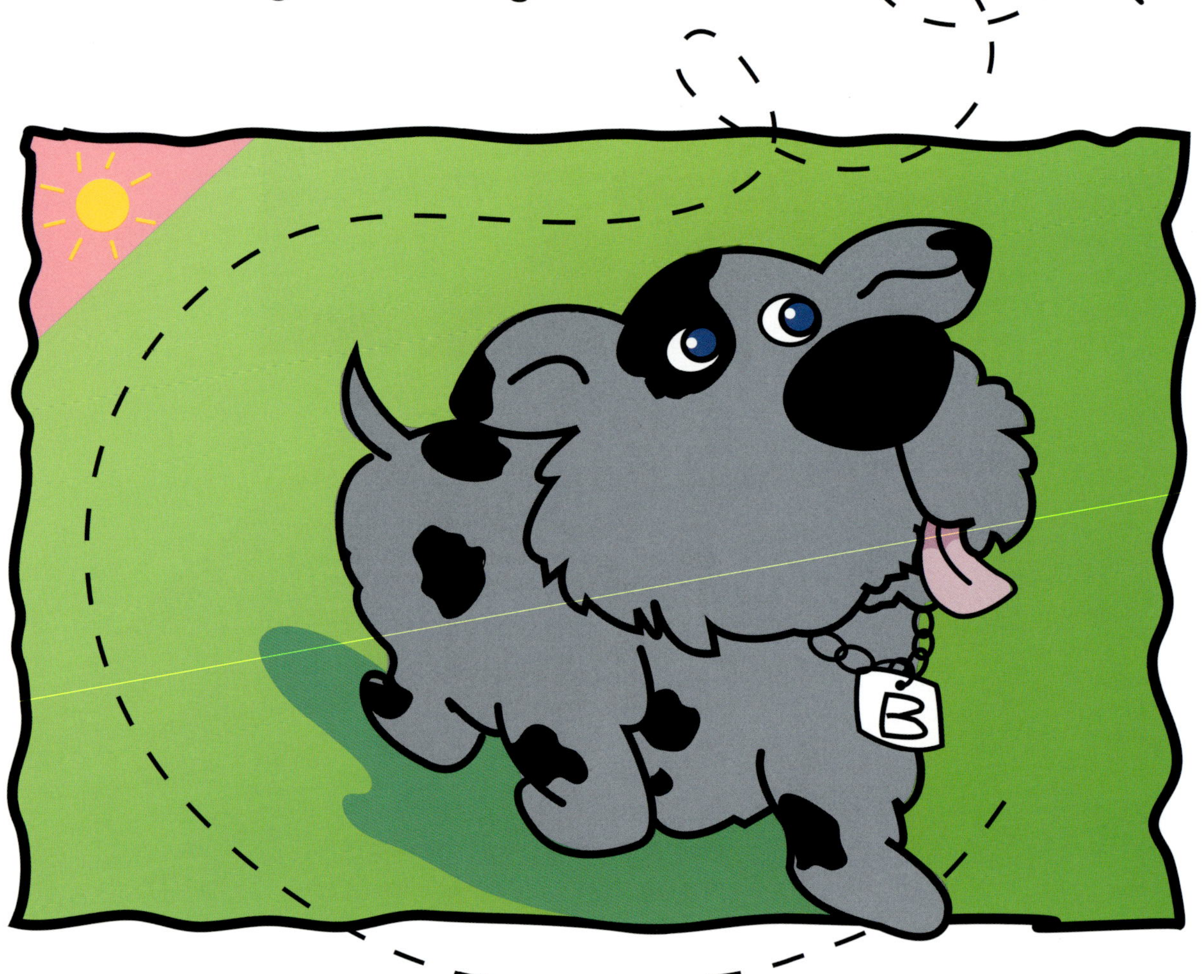

My dog Bunker and I love to go to the park on sunny days.

He likes to chase butterflies and I like to go on the swings.

2

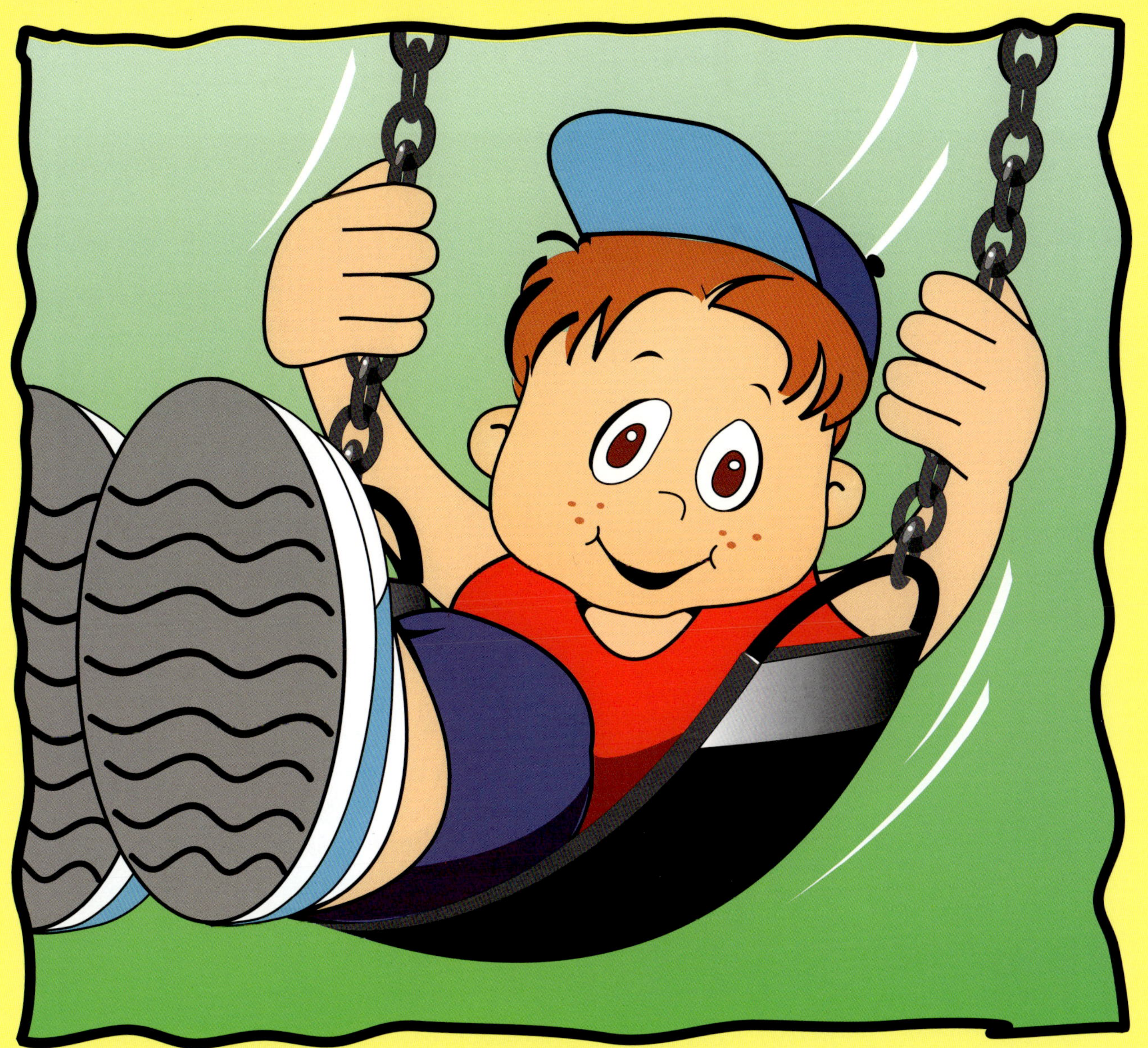

3

One day, my mom took us to the park.
Wheee...swinging high was so much fun!

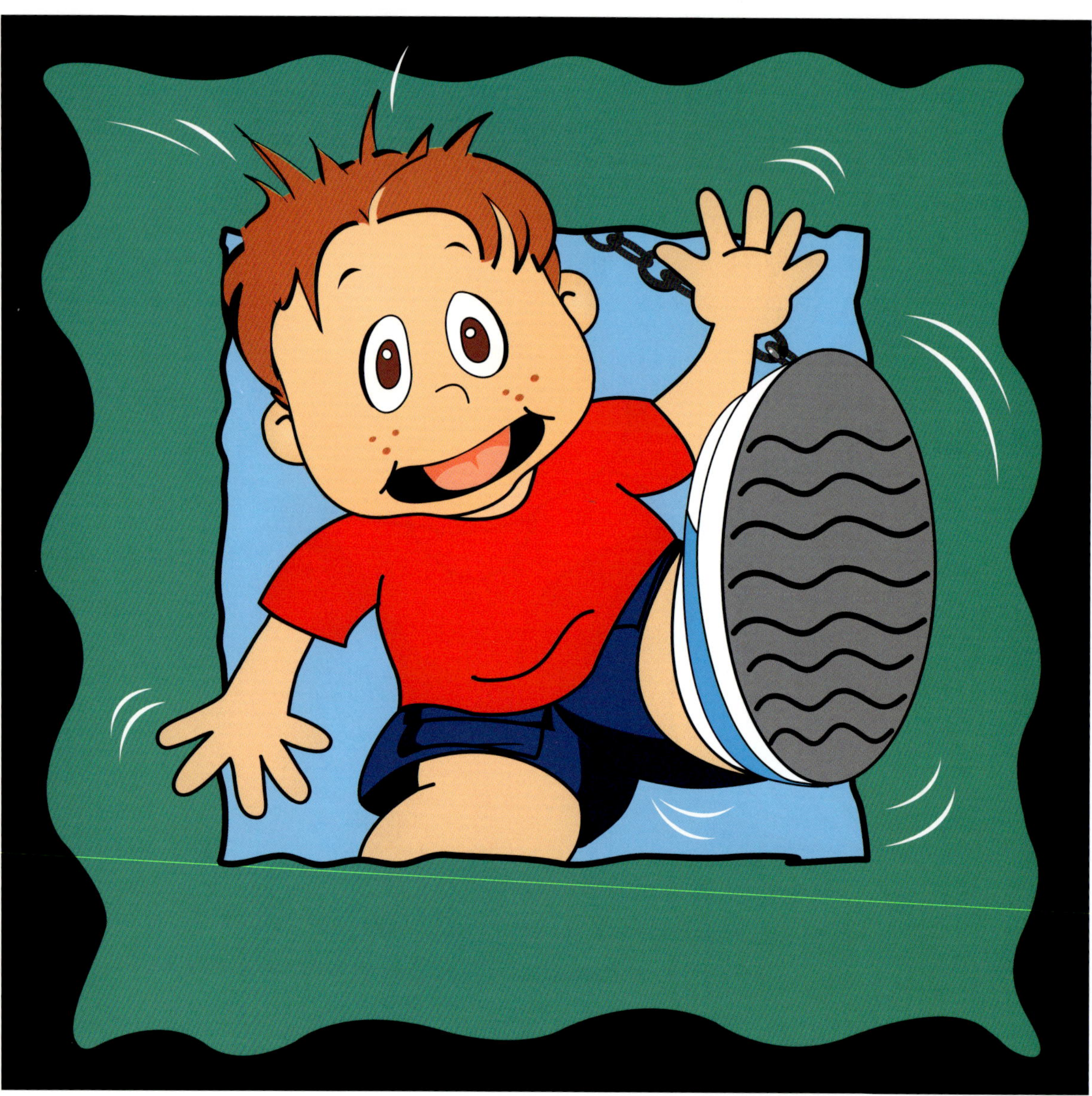

4

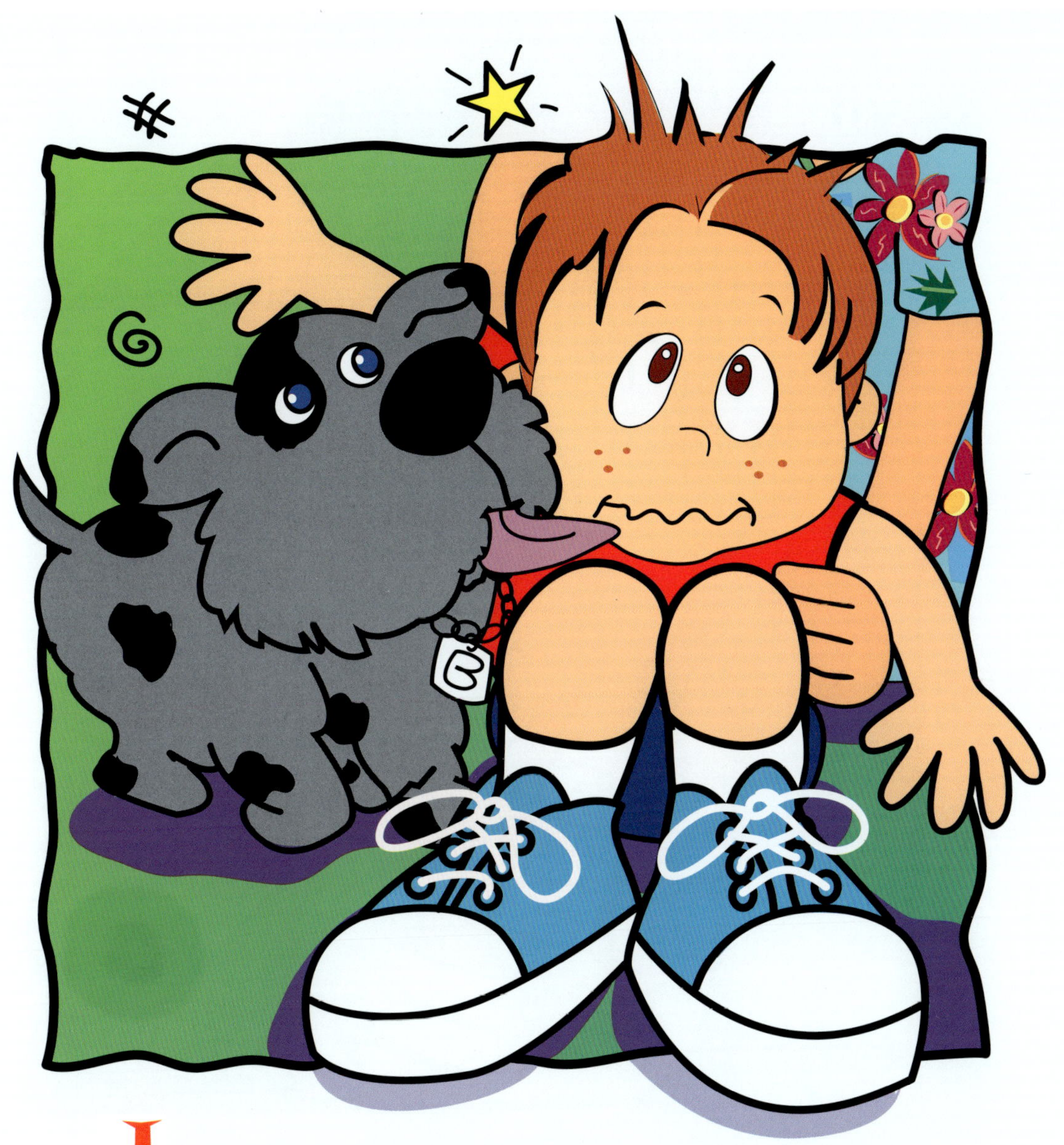

I fell off the swing and hurt my hand. Bunker came running to see if I was OK. My mom said I had better go to the doctor to get my hand checked!

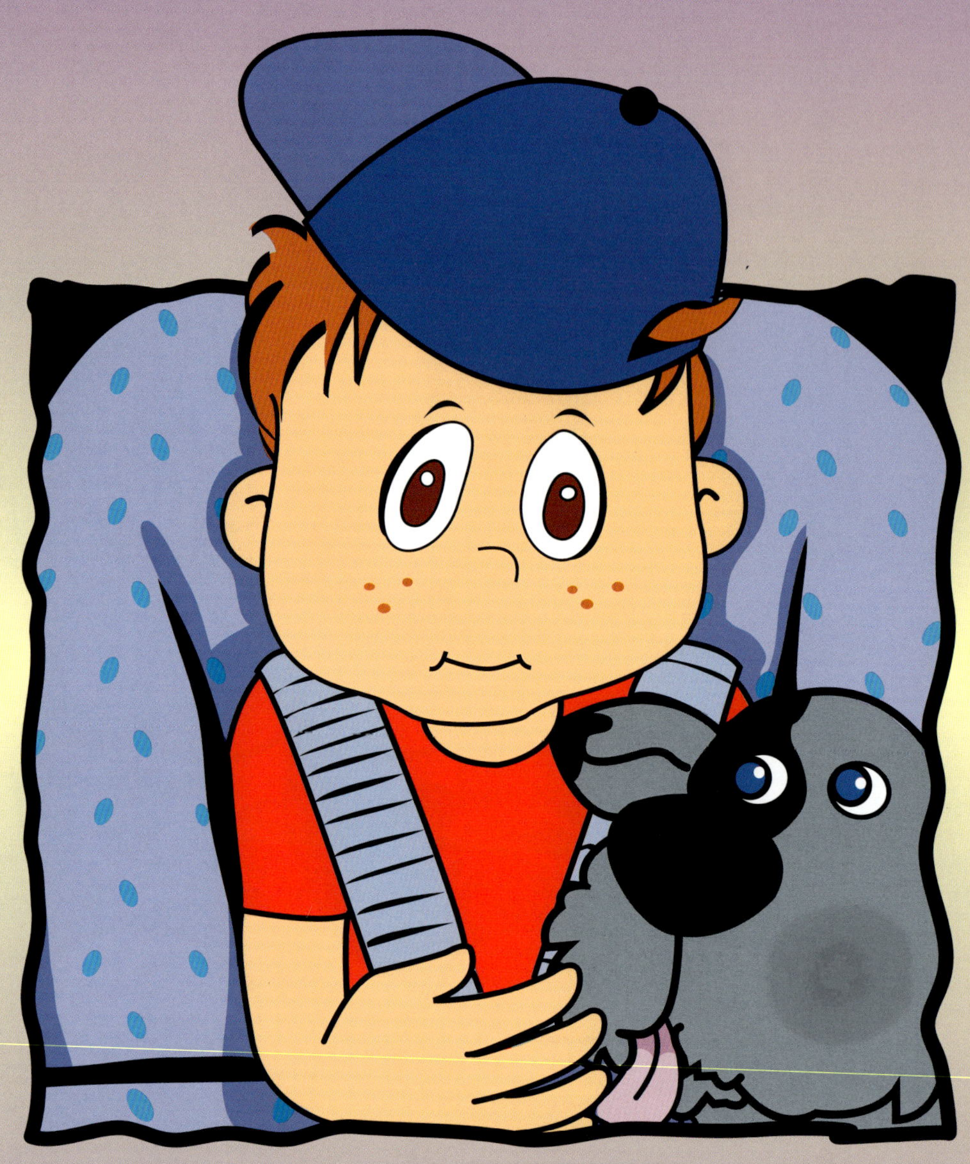

We drove to the doctor's office right away.

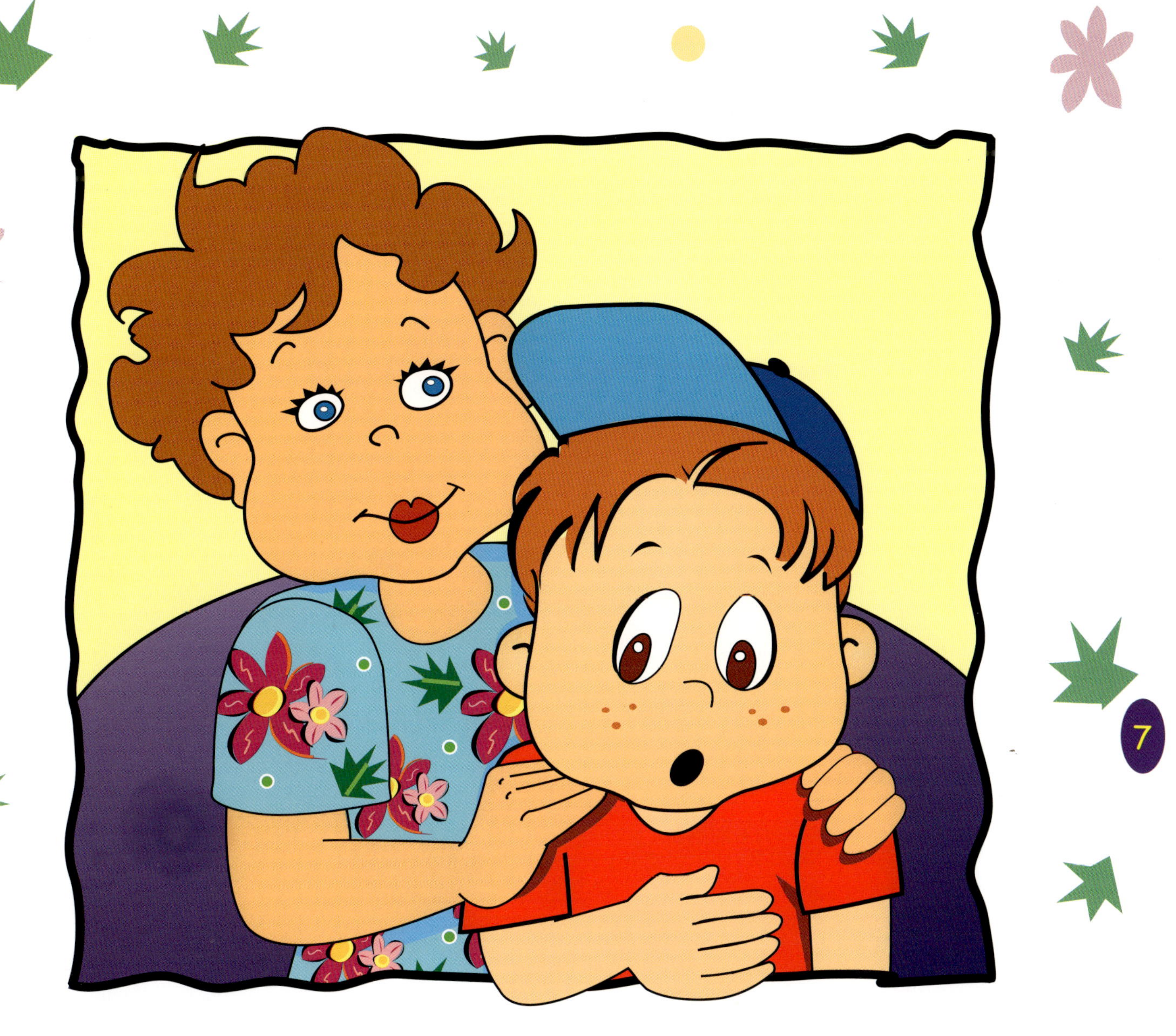

My mom and I had to wait our turn to see the doctor.

Ow…my hand REALLY hurt.

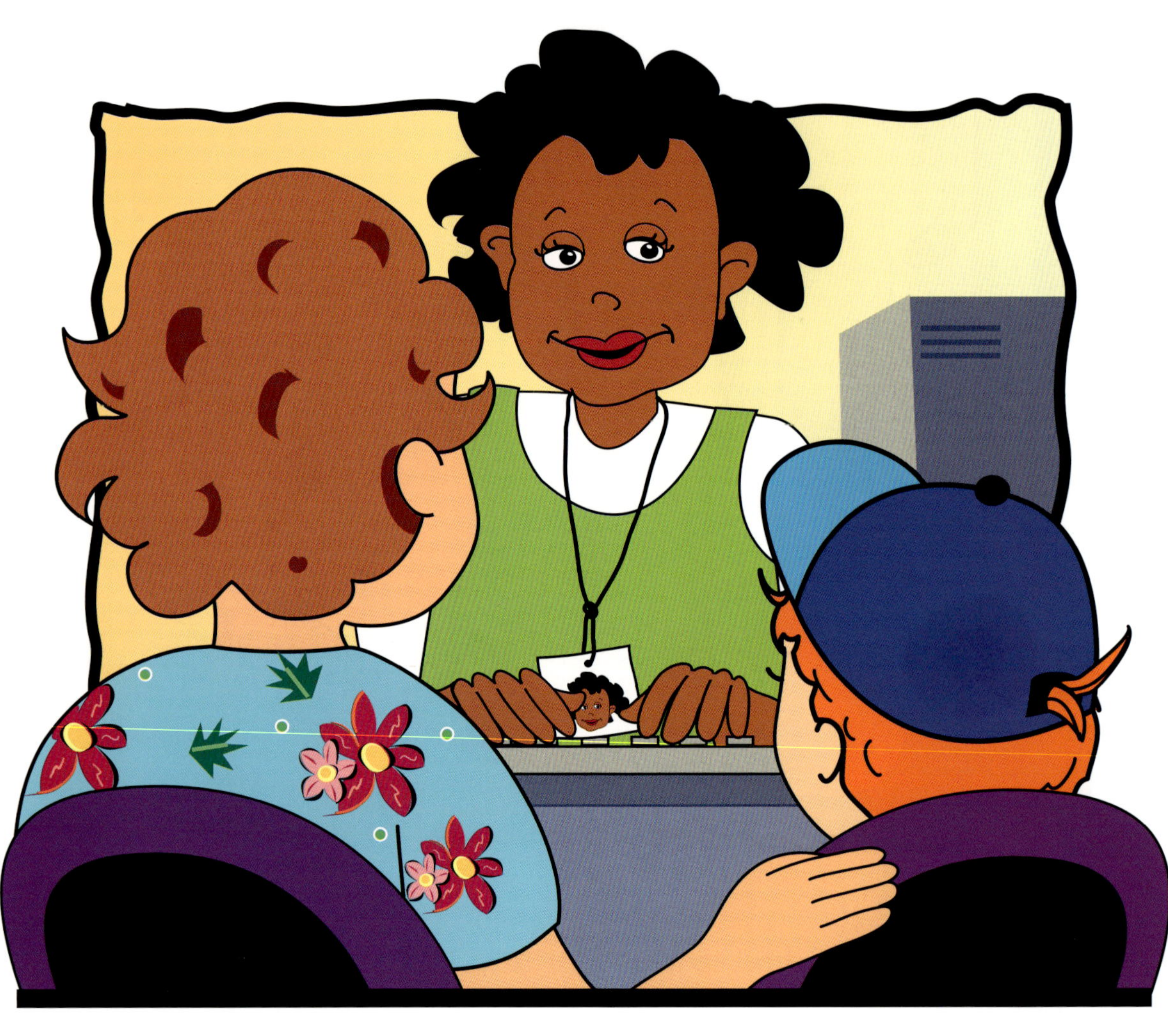

While we waited, a nice lady asked my mom lots of questions. I told her my name was Cooper and that I hoped the doctor would make my hand feel better.

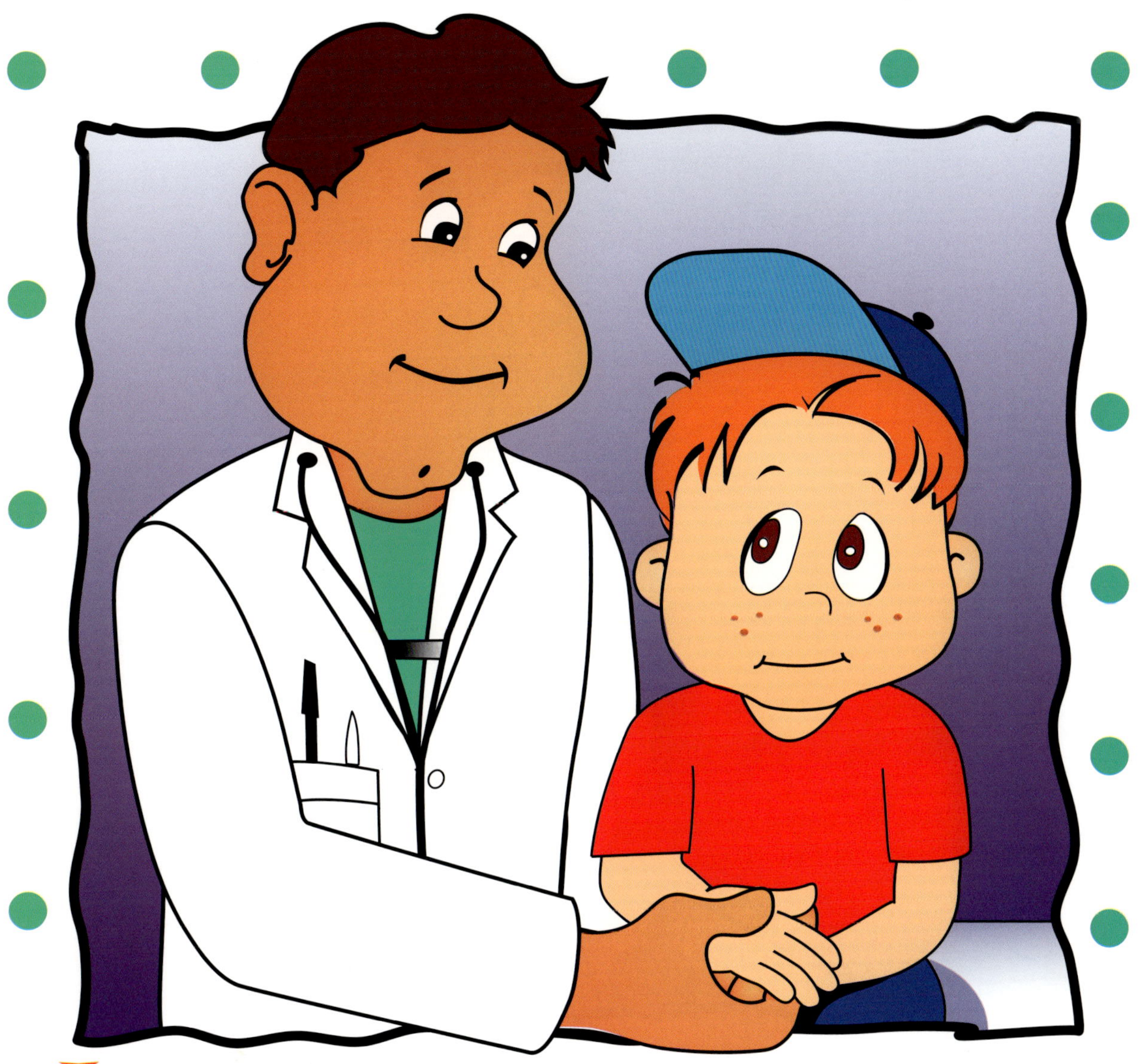

After a little while, they called my name and it was my turn to see the doctor. He was very gentle when he was checking my hand.

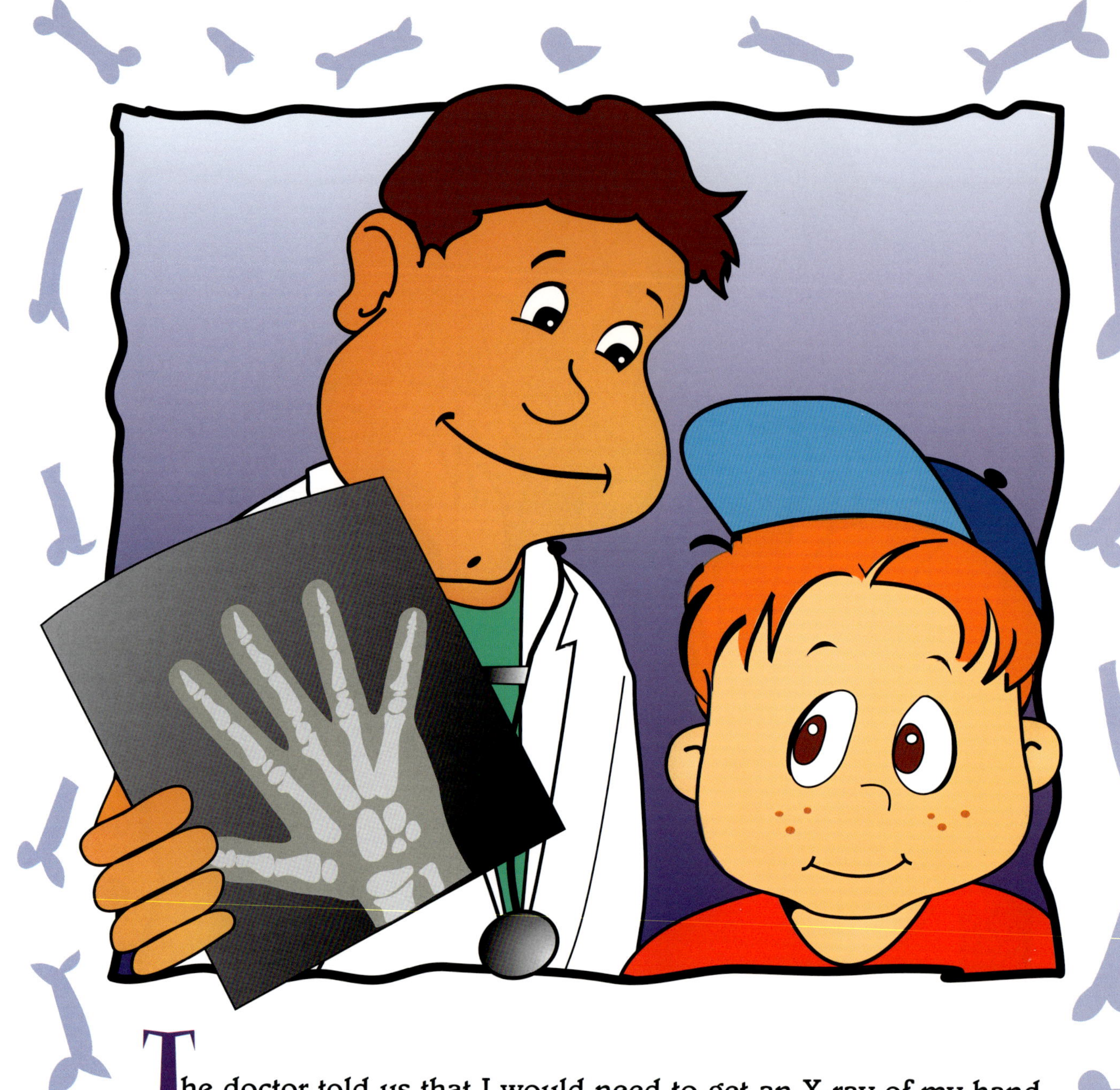

The doctor told us that I would need to get an X-ray of my hand.
He said that an X-ray is a picture of the inside of your body.
An X-ray lets the doctor see if any bones are broken.

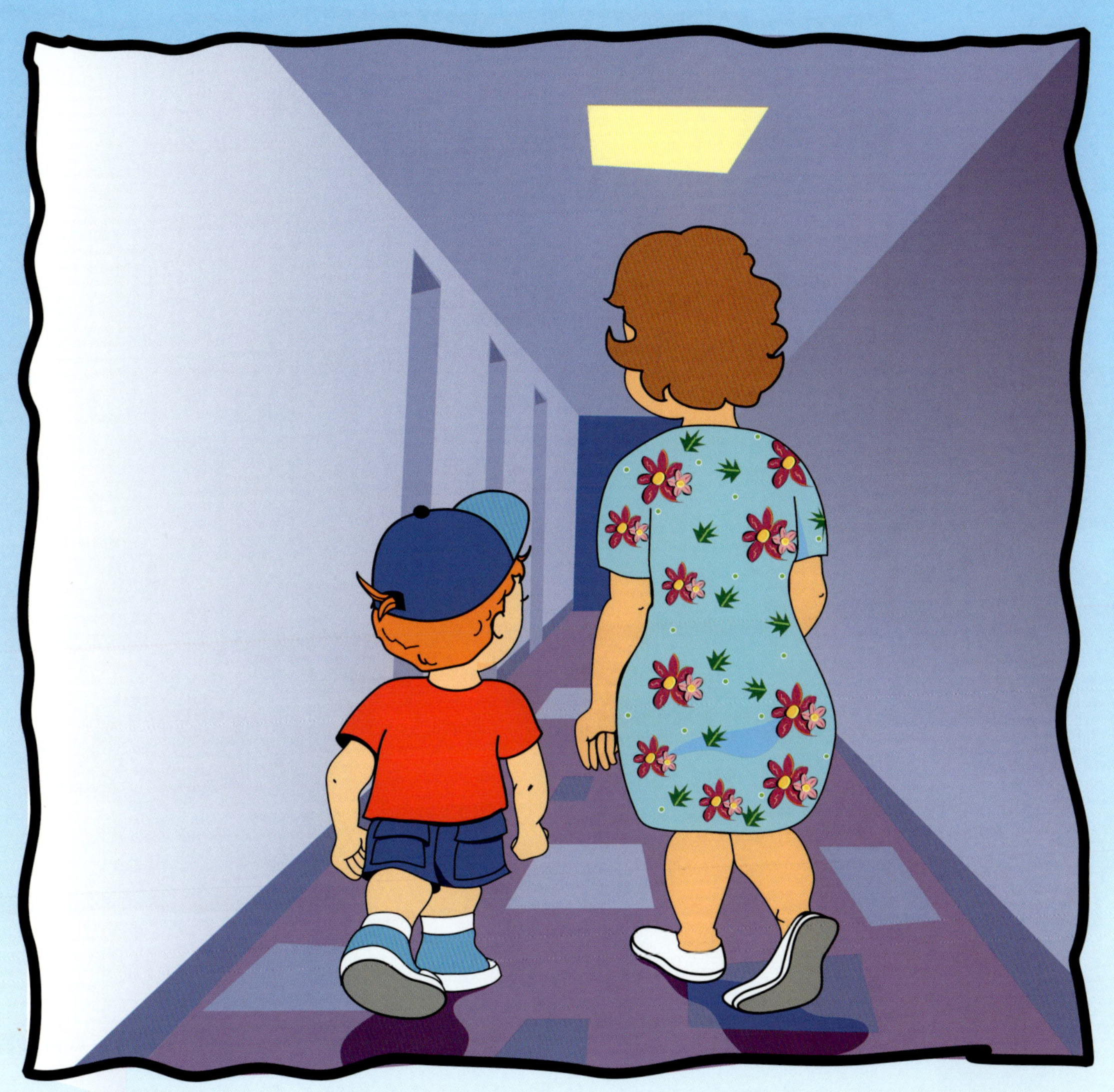

So we left the doctor's office and went to the X-ray room.

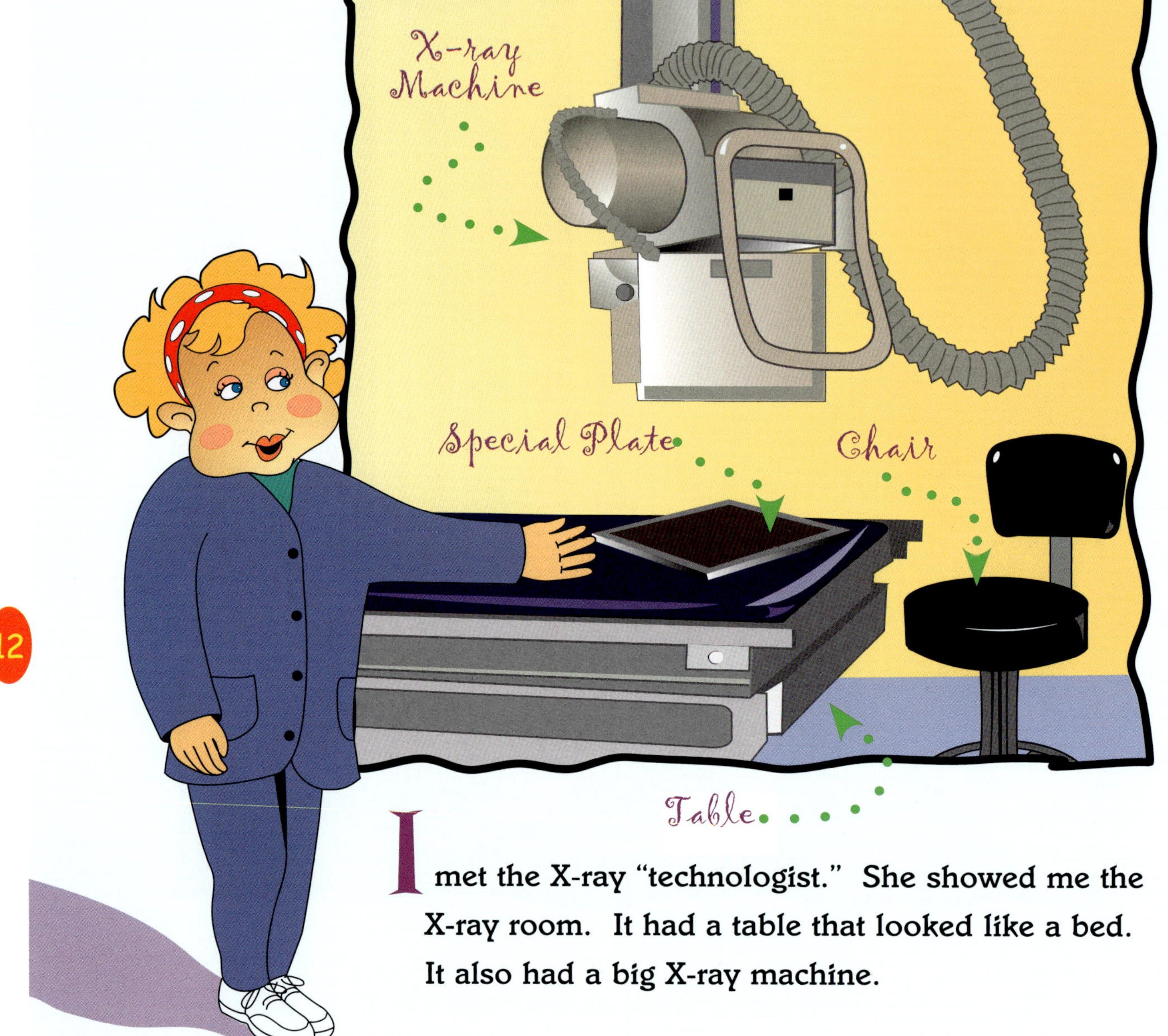

I met the X-ray "technologist." She showed me the X-ray room. It had a table that looked like a bed. It also had a big X-ray machine.

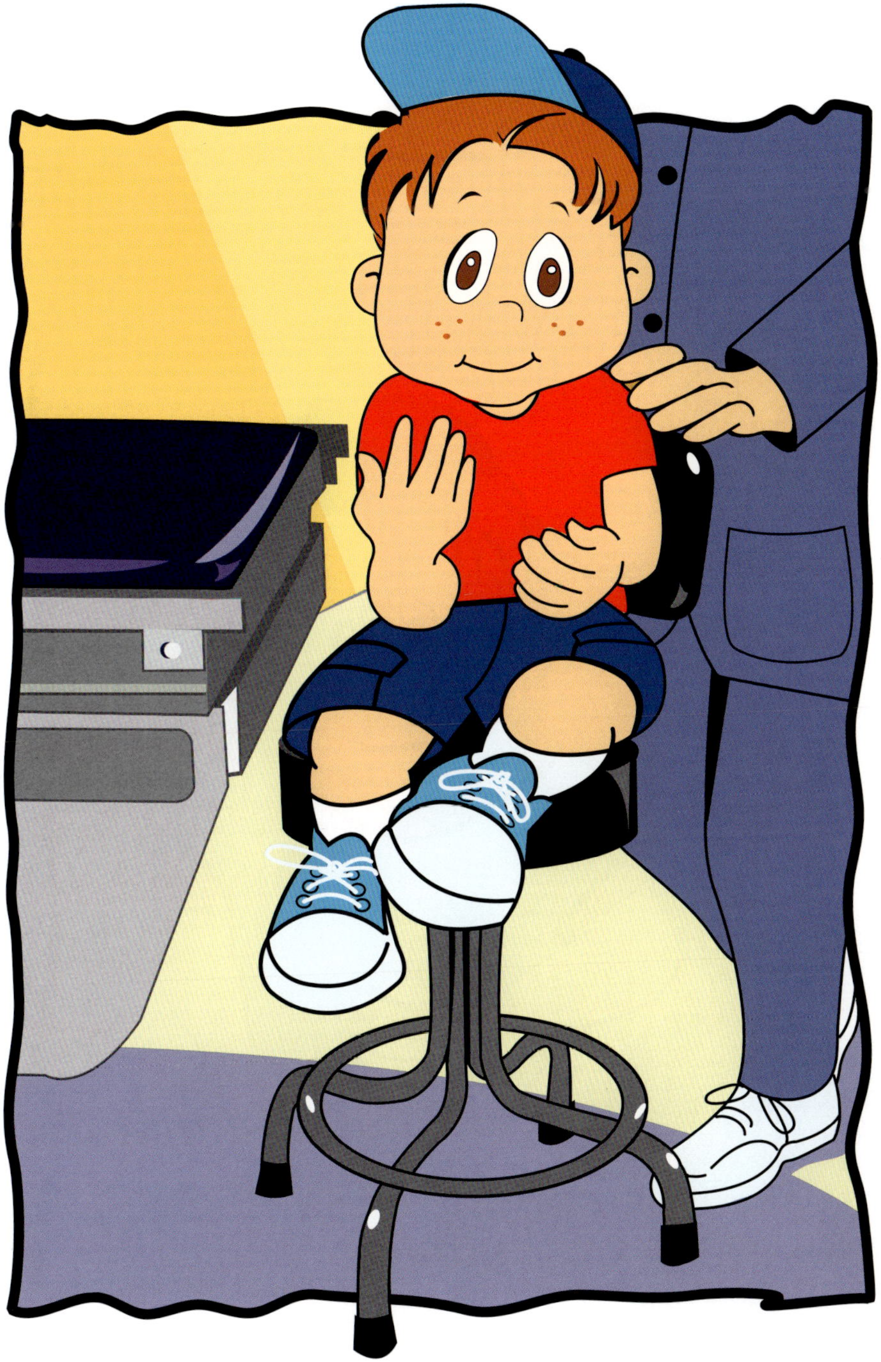

She helped me onto a chair at the end of the table and then showed me what was going to happen.

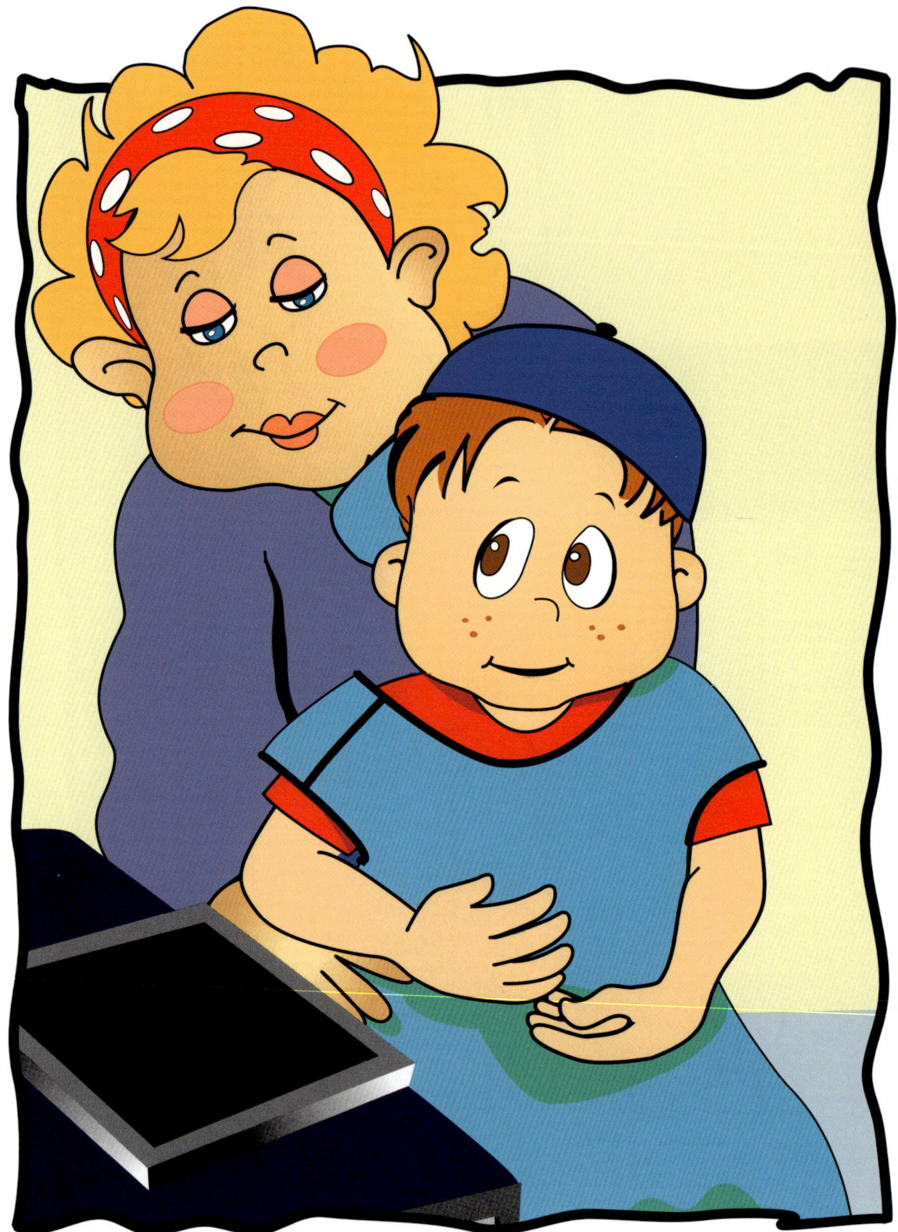

The technologist put a special kind of apron on me. She said it was going to be heavy, but it wasn't TOO heavy for ME!

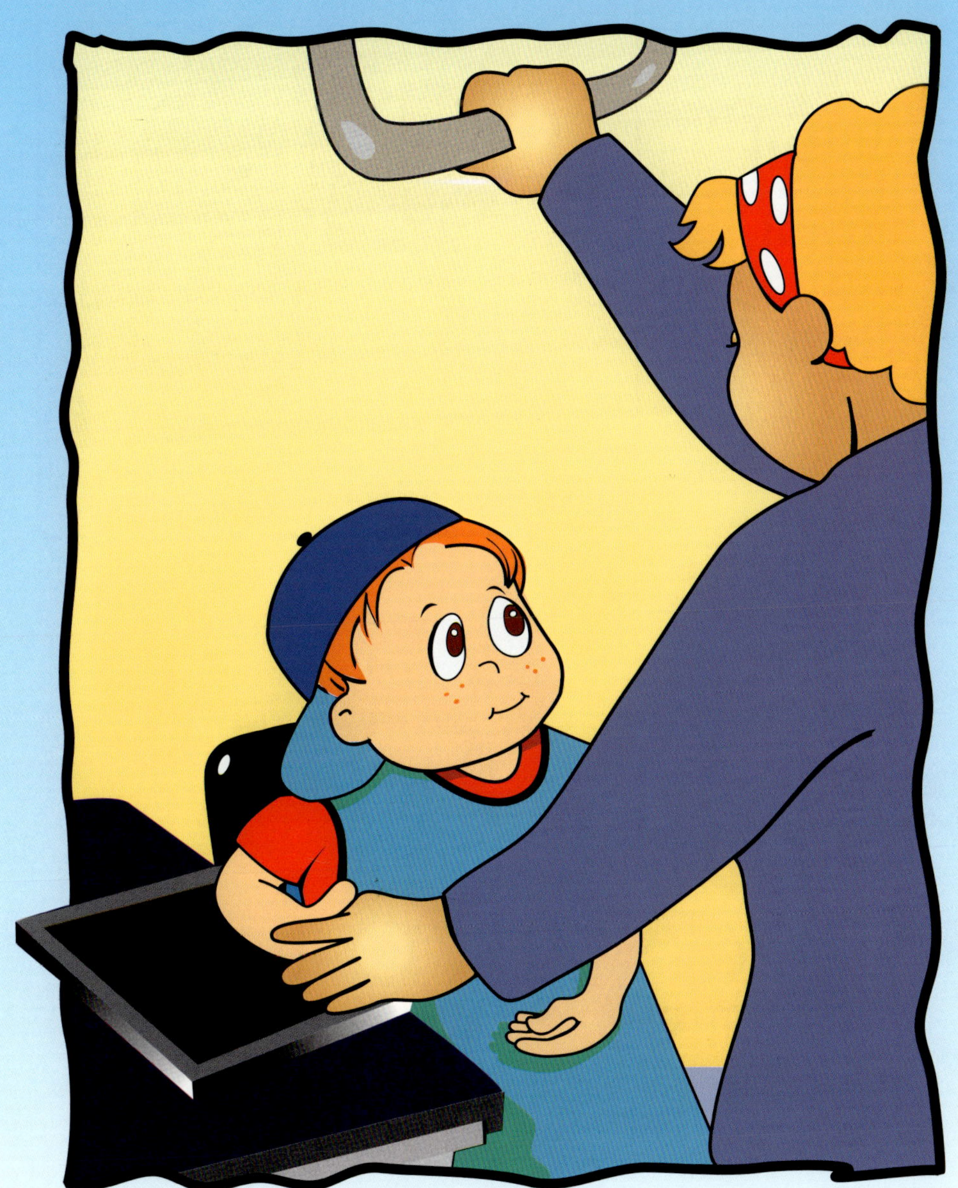

She showed me how the X-ray machine goes up and down, and back and forth to get the best pictures of my hand.

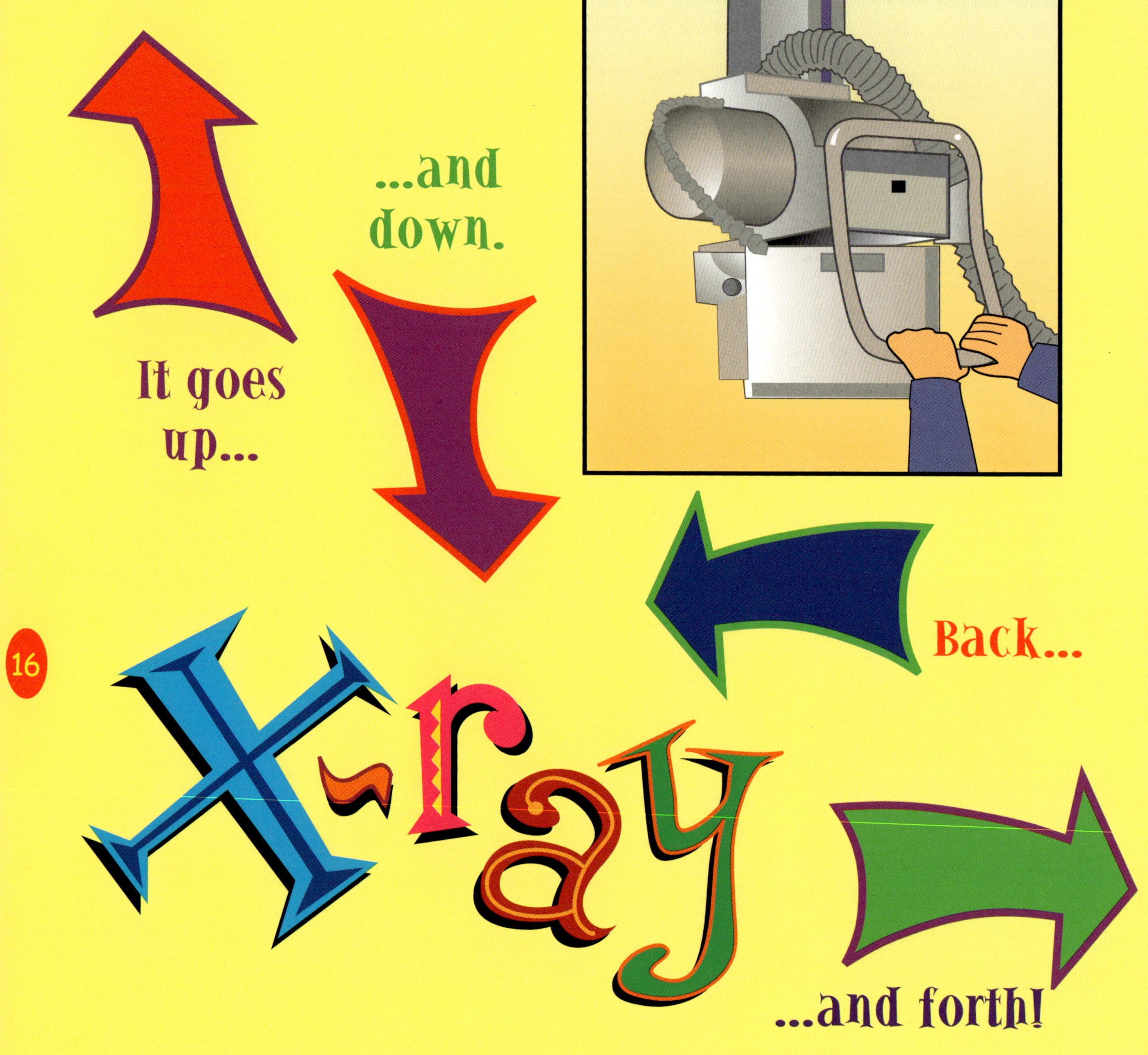
It goes up...
...and down.
Back...
...and forth!
X-ray

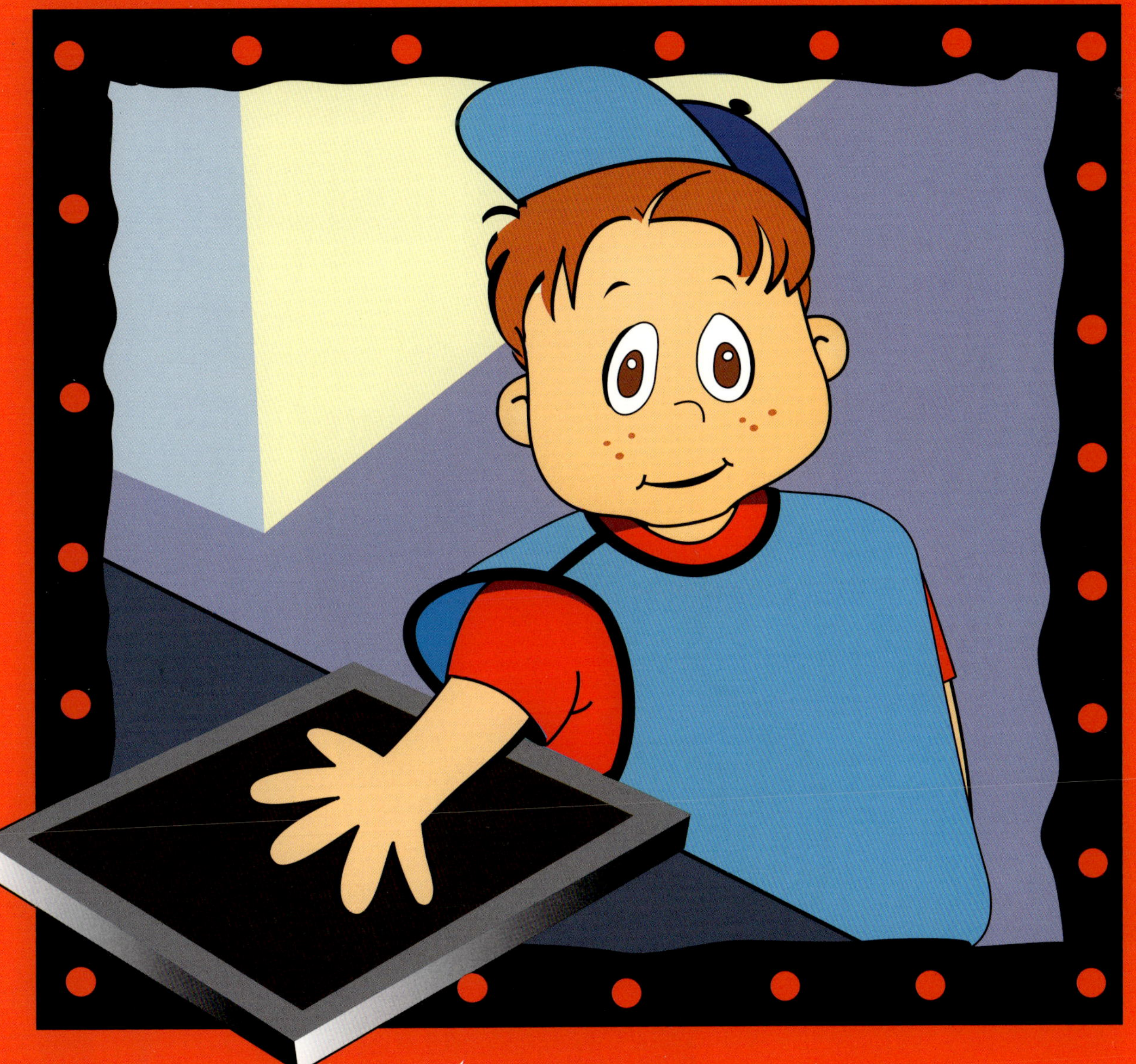

She put my hand on a special plate and
told me to hold my hand very still.

There was a
special light

shining

down on
my hand.

18

It was
like a big

flashlight.

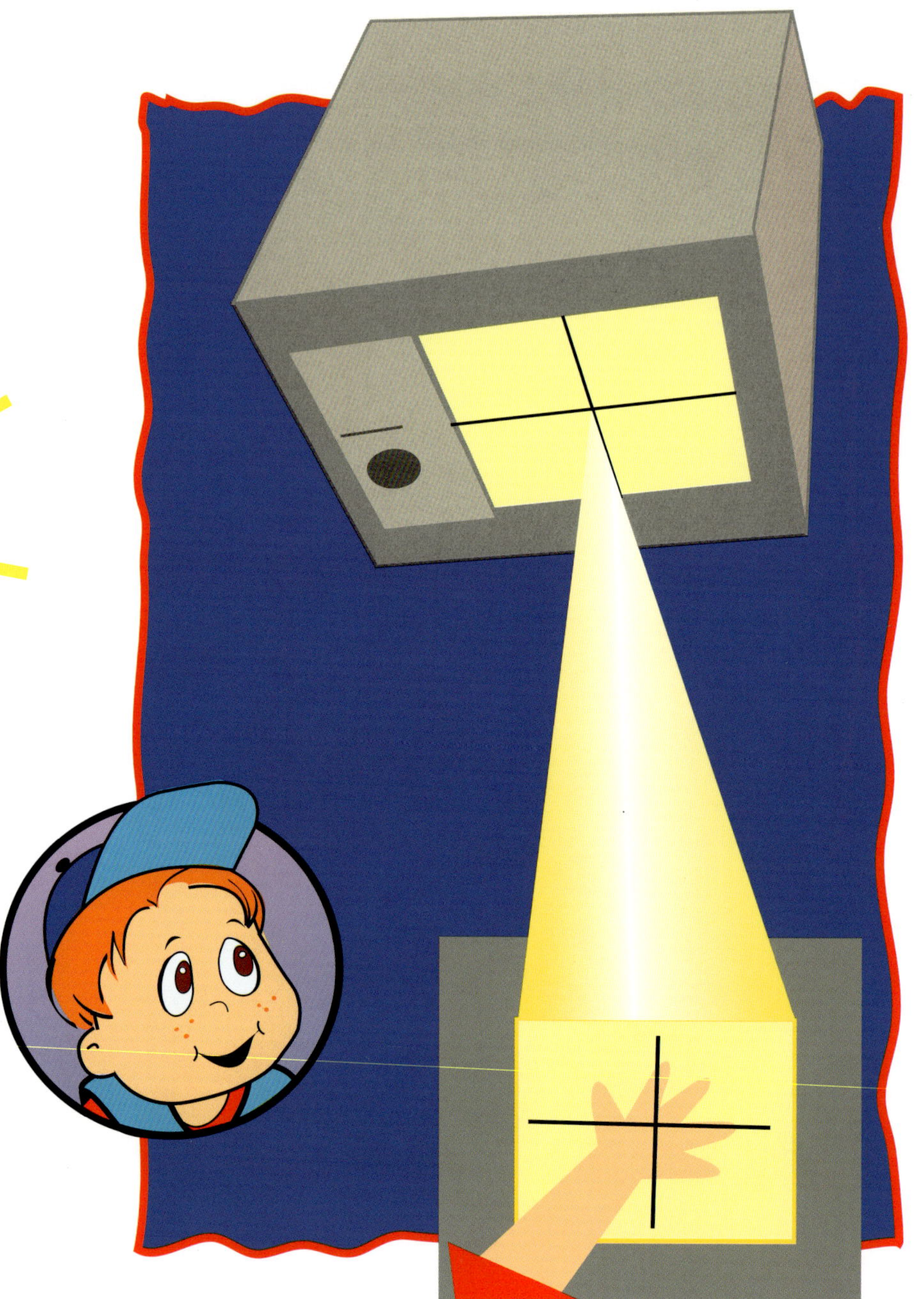

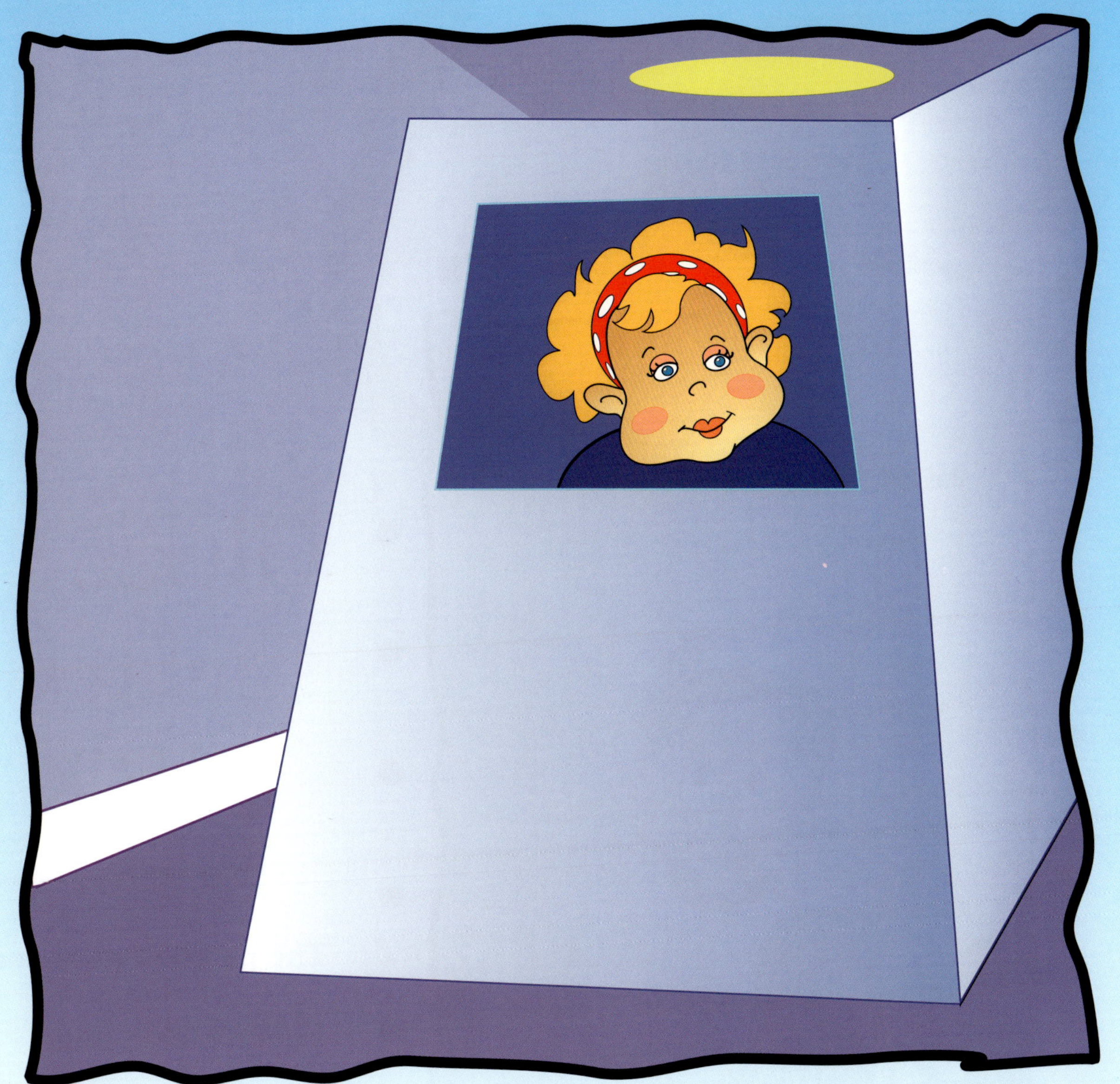

Then the technologist went behind a wall to take the X-ray pictures. I could see her through a glass window. She smiled at me.

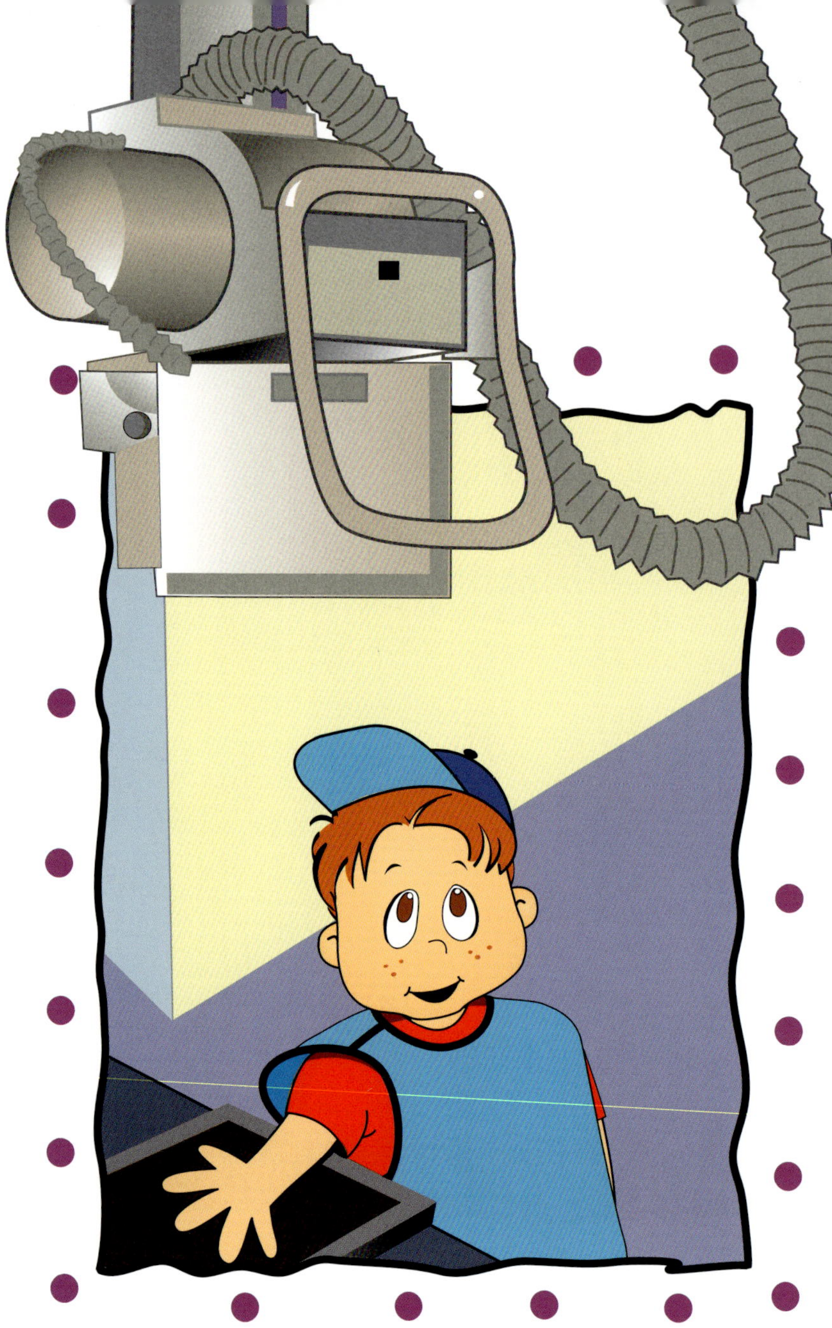

Click...
...click...
CLICK

The pictures were done.

I hadn't felt a thing!

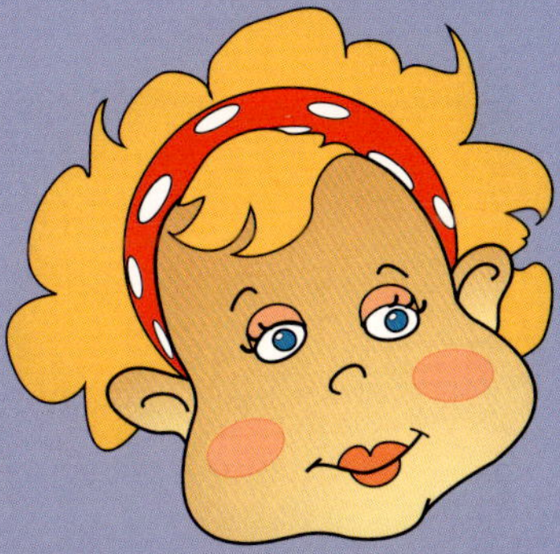

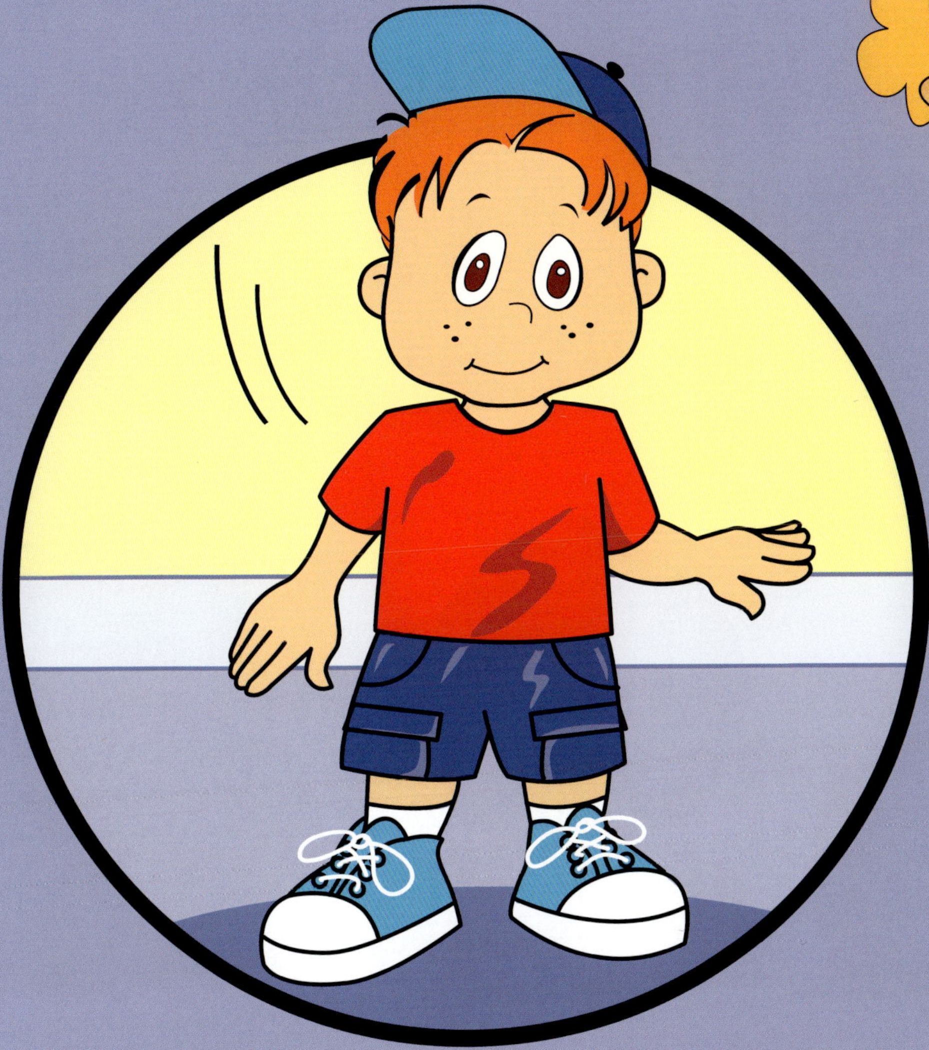

The technologist helped me down from the chair.

She thanked me for holding so still…I told her it was EASY!

21

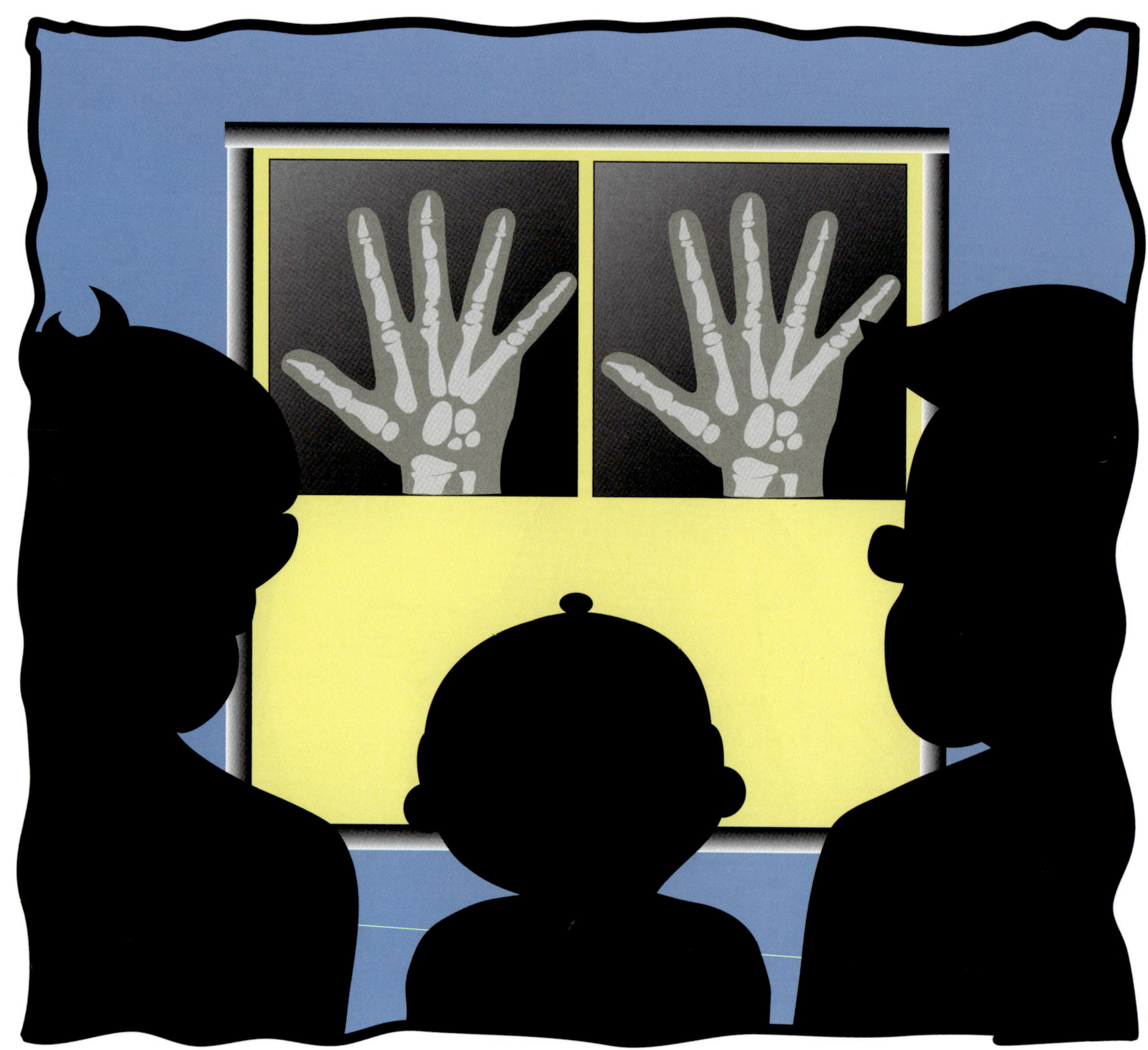

We went back to the doctor's office and he showed us the
X-ray pictures on a light box. The light box was bright
and helped us to see the bones inside my hand.

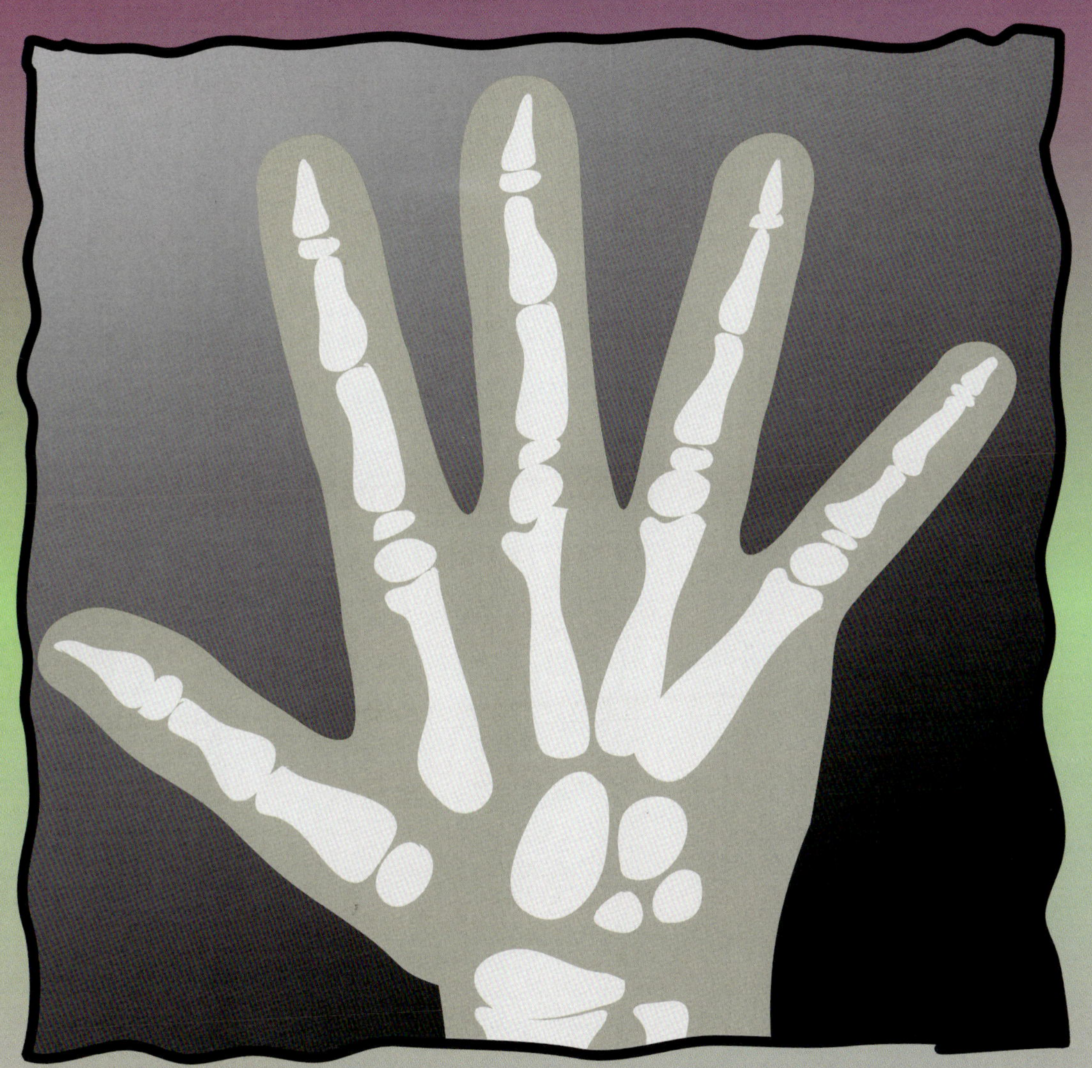

The doctor said he didn't see any broken bones.

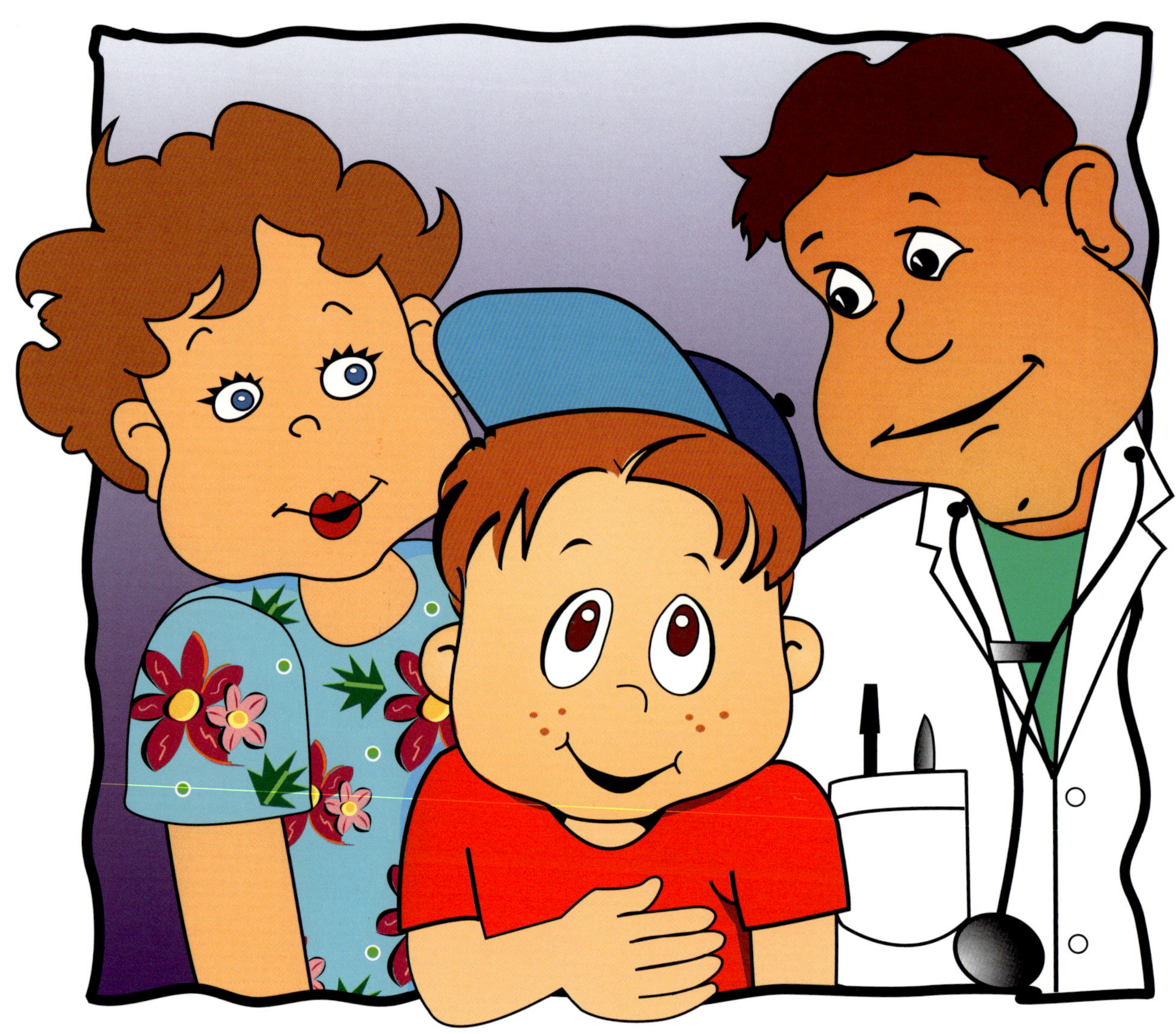

The doctor told me that my hand would be just fine. It would be a little sore for awhile, but it would get better.

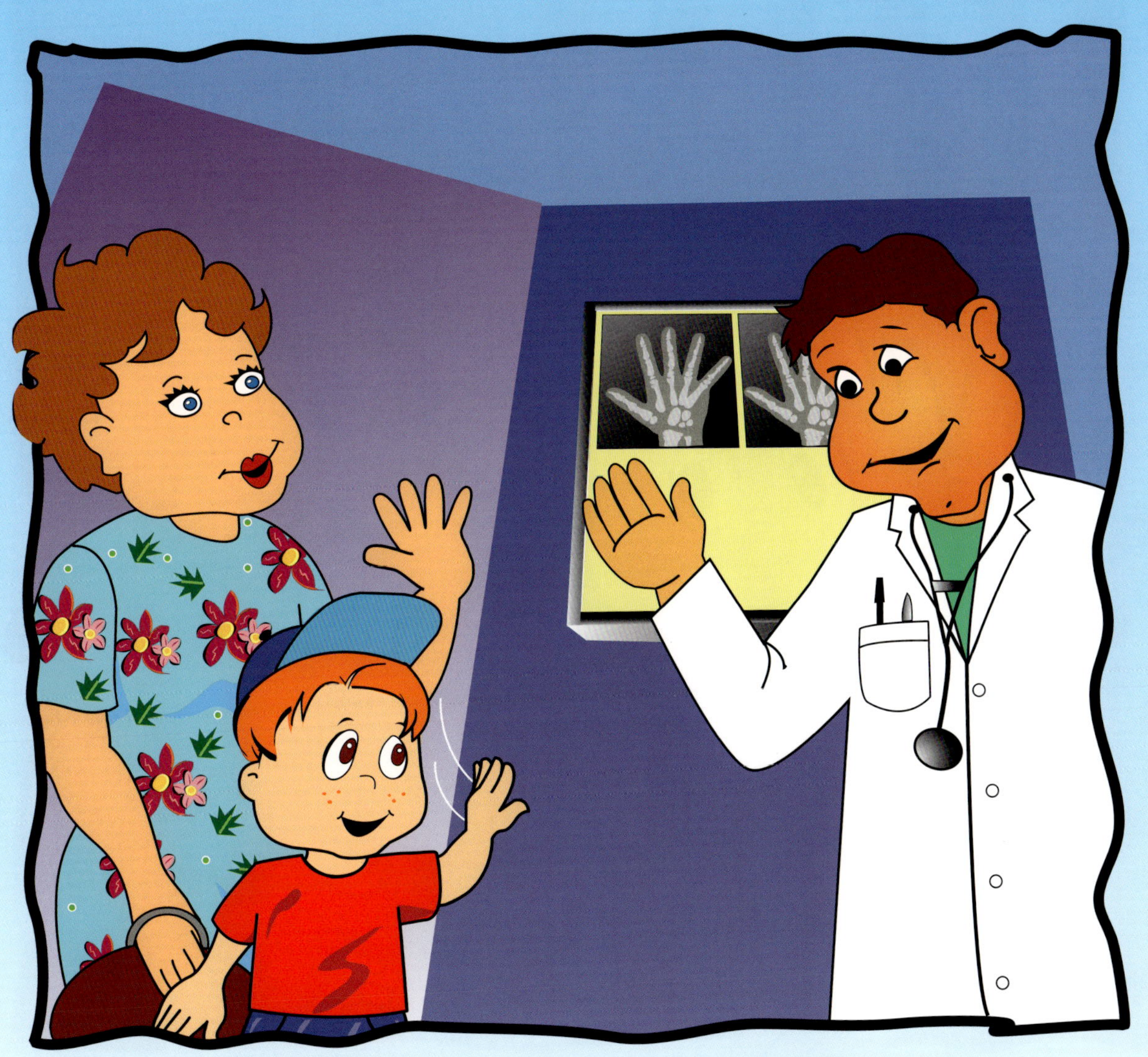

We said goodbye to the doctor and went home.

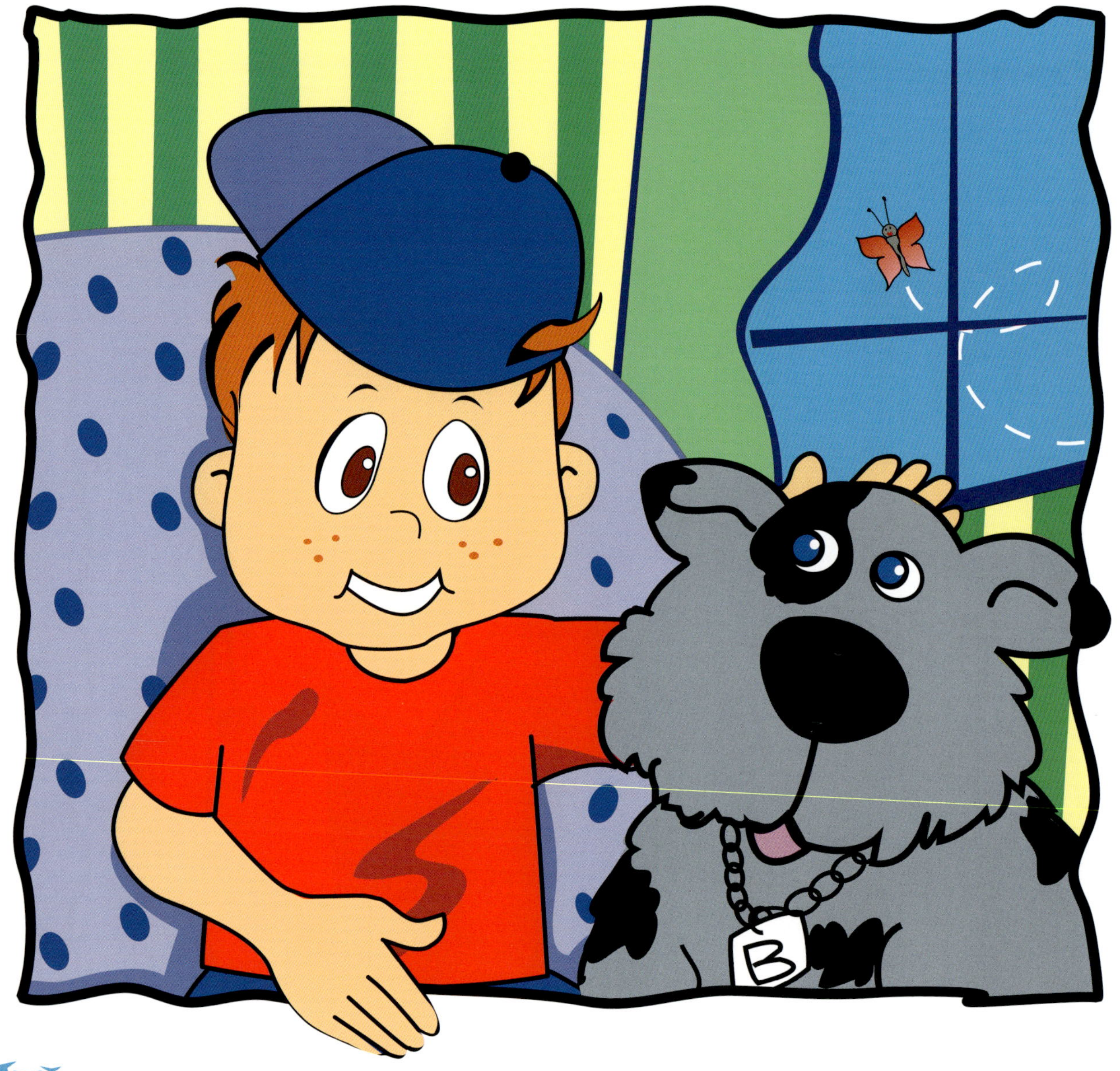

When we got home, I told Bunker all about the doctor and my X-ray pictures.

Can you remember what happened to Cooper in the X-ray room?

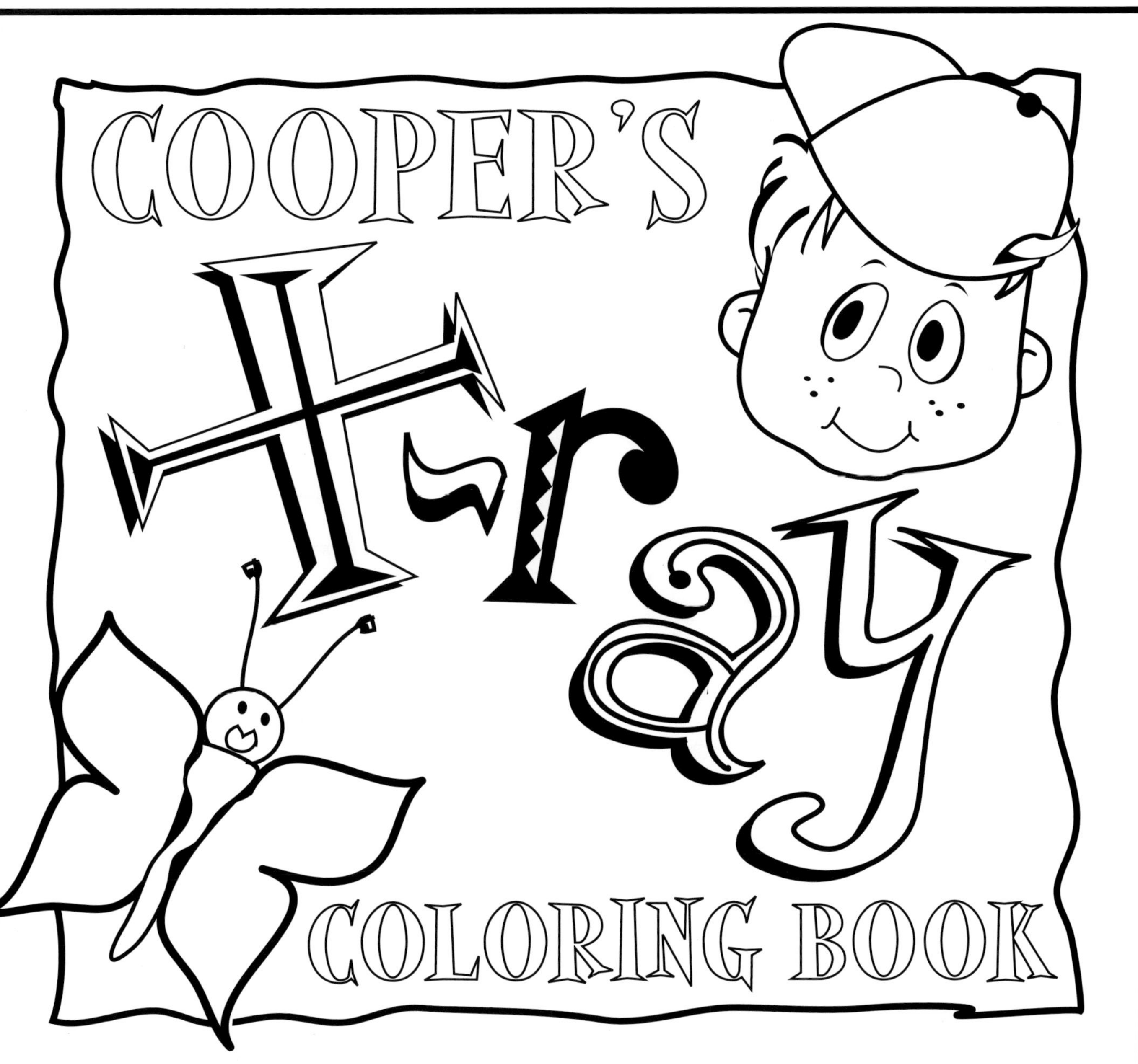
COOPER'S
X-ray
COLORING BOOK
27

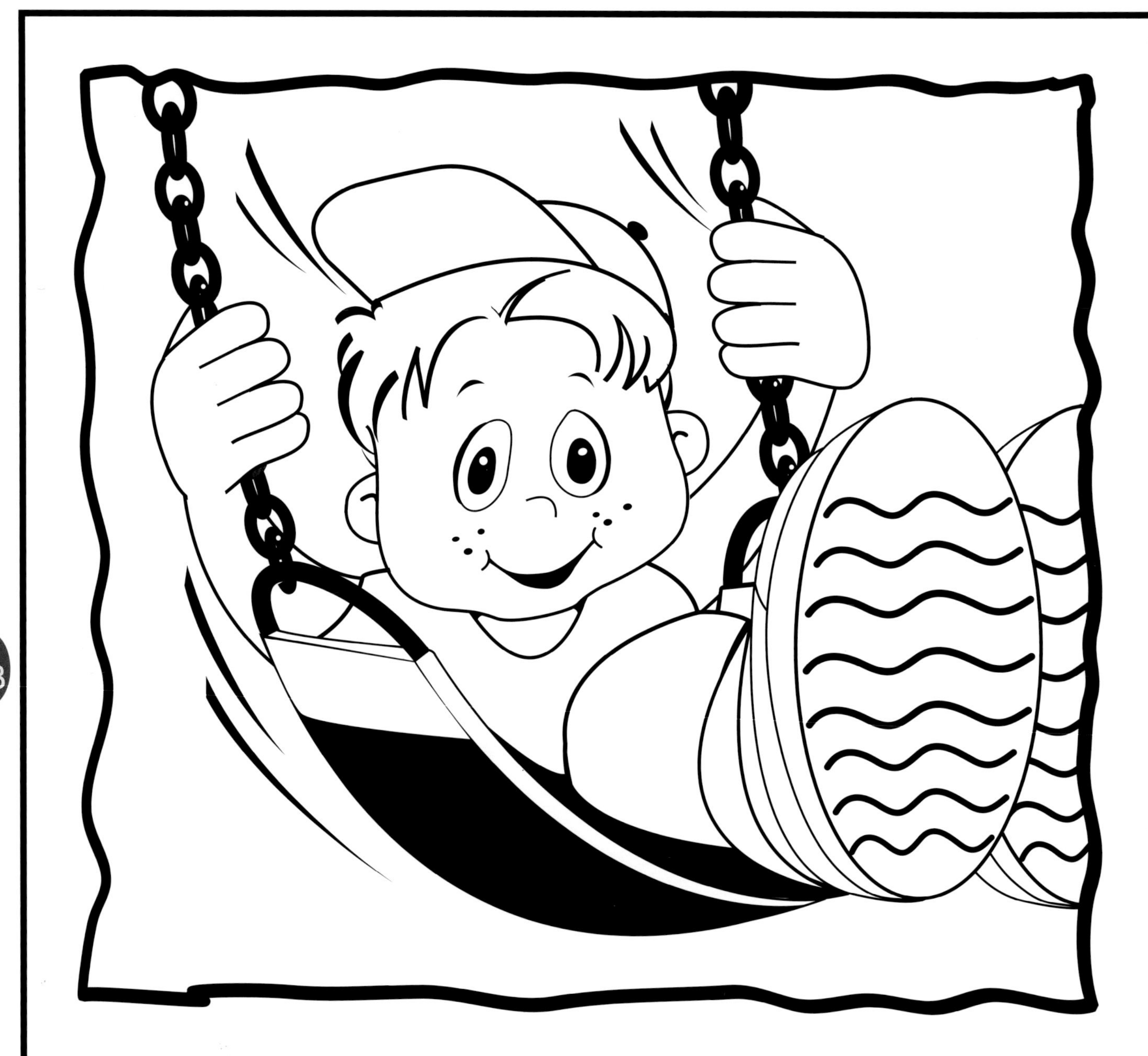

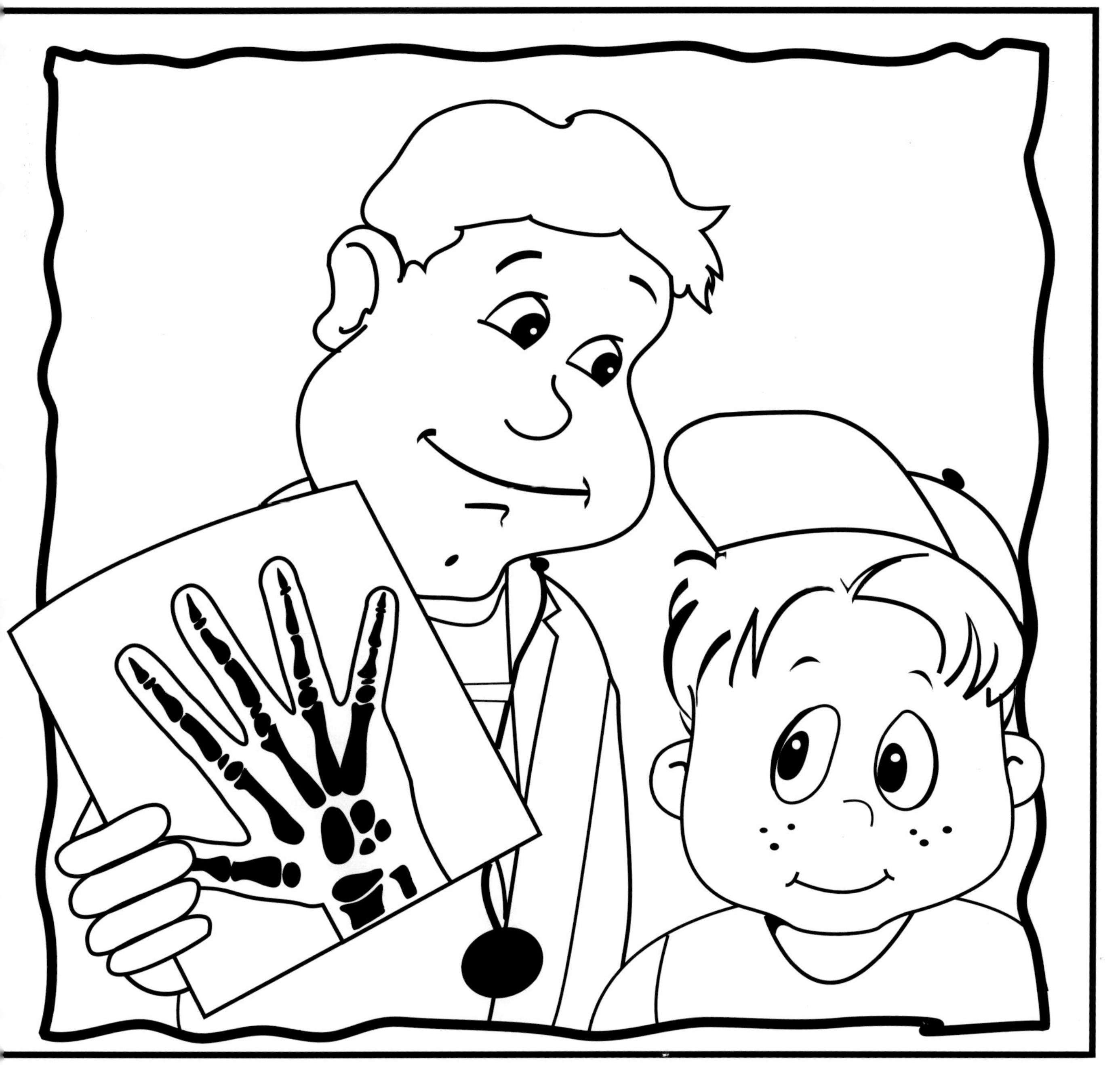

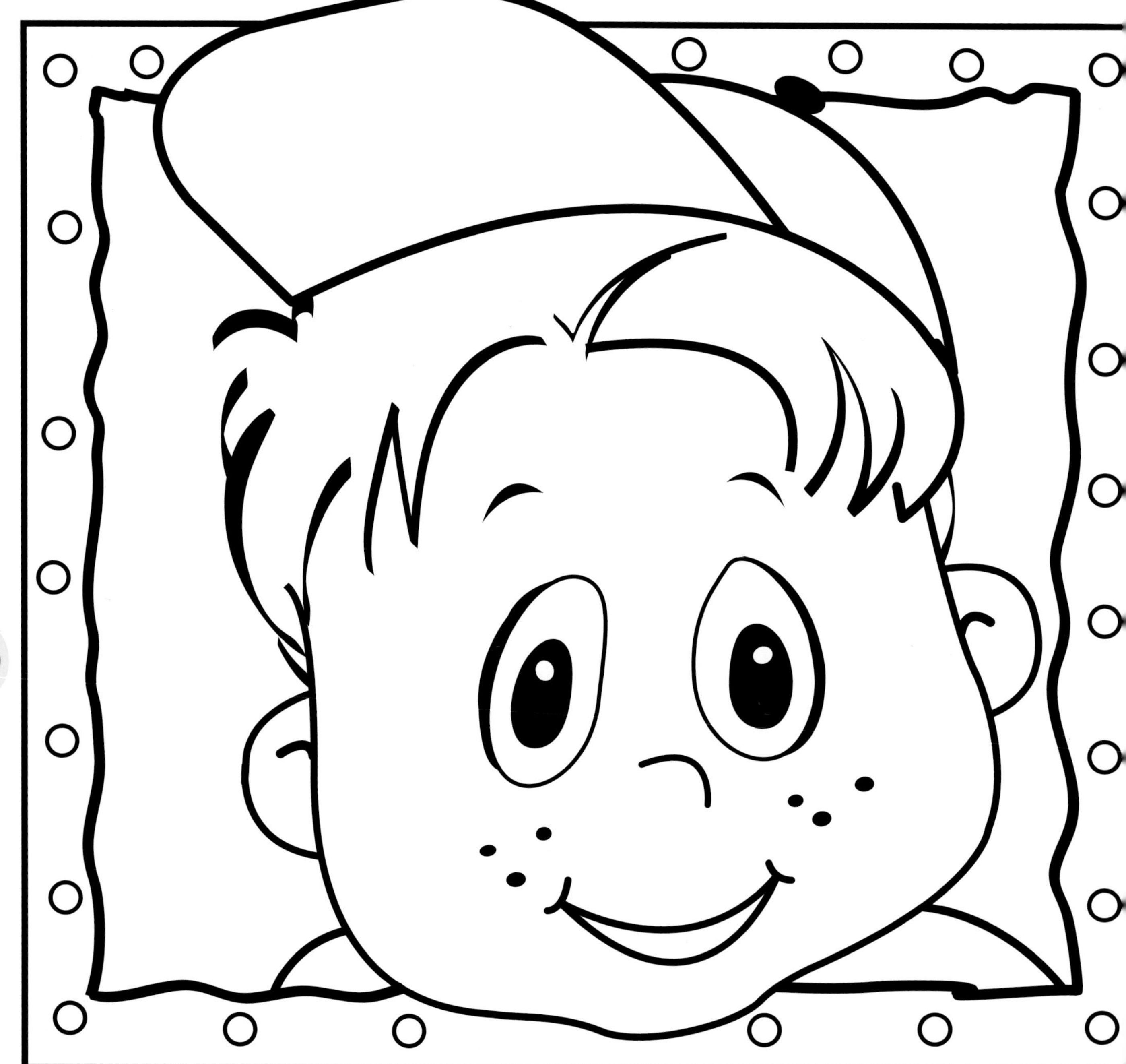

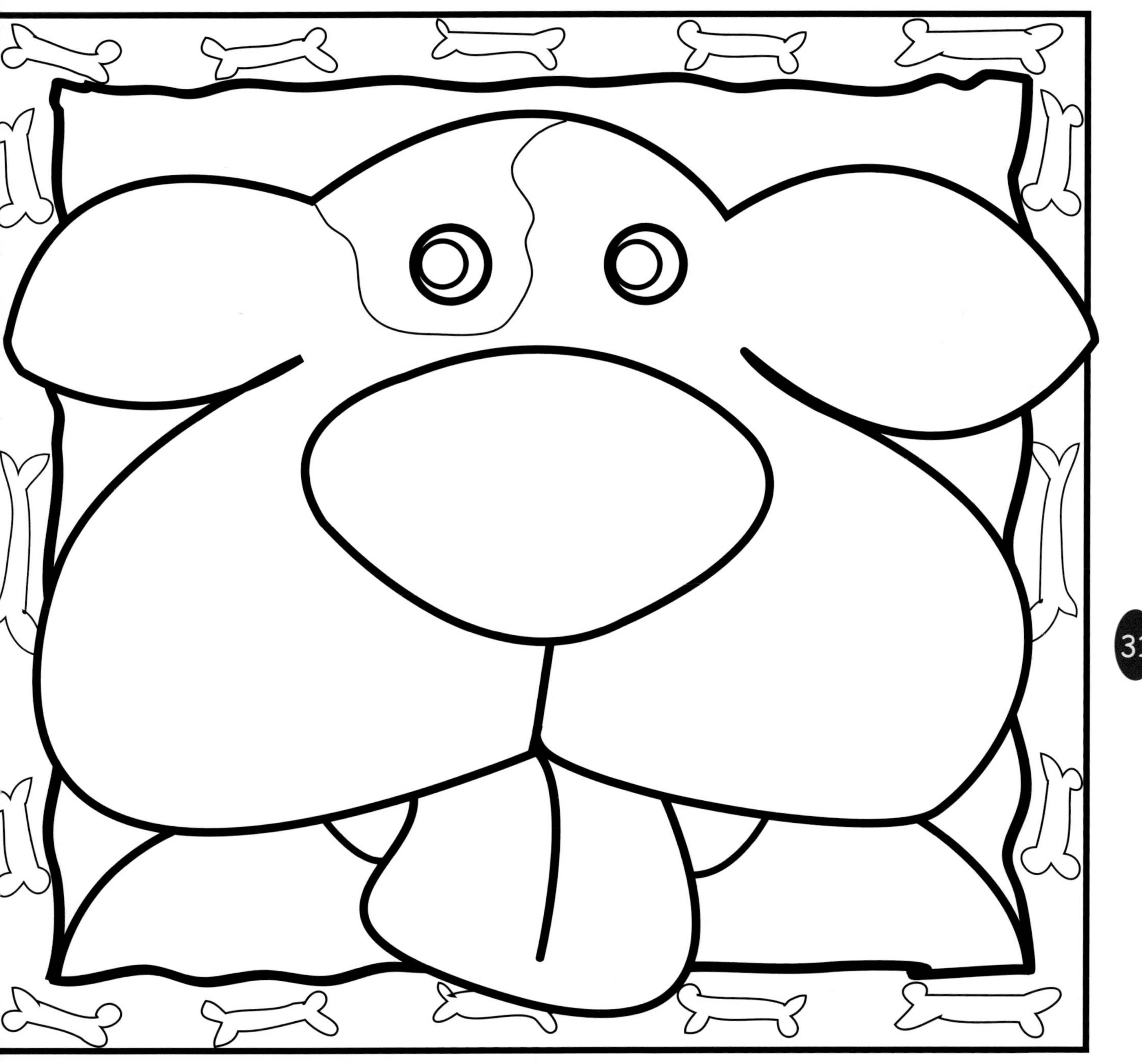

Cast of Characters